THE ACCESSIBLE GUIDE
TO FLORENCE

THE ACCESSIBLE

GUIDE TO FLORENCE

Cornelia Danielson

To order additional copies of this book, contact:
Xlibris Corporation
1-888-795-4274
www.Xlibris.com
Orders@Xlibris.com
23692

CONTENTS

Acknowledgments

Writing a guide describing accessibility in a Renaissance city was, to say the least, a challenge, an ambitious project with countless stones to unturn. Without the overwhelming cooperation and courtesy extended to Barrier Free Travel on the part of the directors and personnel of the museums, hotels, restaurants, theaters, transportation systems, and countless other organizations in the city of Florence who allowed us to inspect, measure, and evaluate their properties, this project would not have been possible. Special thanks are extended to the Florentine public bus transportation agency ATAF for permission to use their excellent plan, and to Maurizio Martini and Valerio Marucelli of Studio Comunica & Associati-Mediaetica for the floor plans, preparation of the maps, and cover photographs. Alessio Focardi, from the CGIL Ufficio Disabili, and Michela Neri, formerly of the Cooperativa 2001, helped to conduct the surveys, giving invaluable insight into a view of the world from wheels. The useful observations of many who have consulted Barrier Free Travel's services, and especially those of Michele DeSha and Howard Chabner of San Francisco who also suggested the inclusion of the glossary and metric conversion table, are scattered throughout the book. Appreciation is also extended to Barrier Free Travel's board members for their time and advice over the five years since the organization was founded. Generous support and encouragement have been given to the project by Mary and Harold Danielson; and Alex and Sebastian Vismara have indirectly contributed from behind the scenes by patiently waiting so many evenings for their mother to emerge from the office to fix their dinner. Certainly without the enthusiasm and ideas of Jennifer Cook, this project may never have gotten off the ground. Final and grateful acknowledgment is due to the Vidda Foundation and especially to Ursula Corning whose generosity brought Italy into the hearts of so many during her lifetime and will continue to do so through the publication of this book.

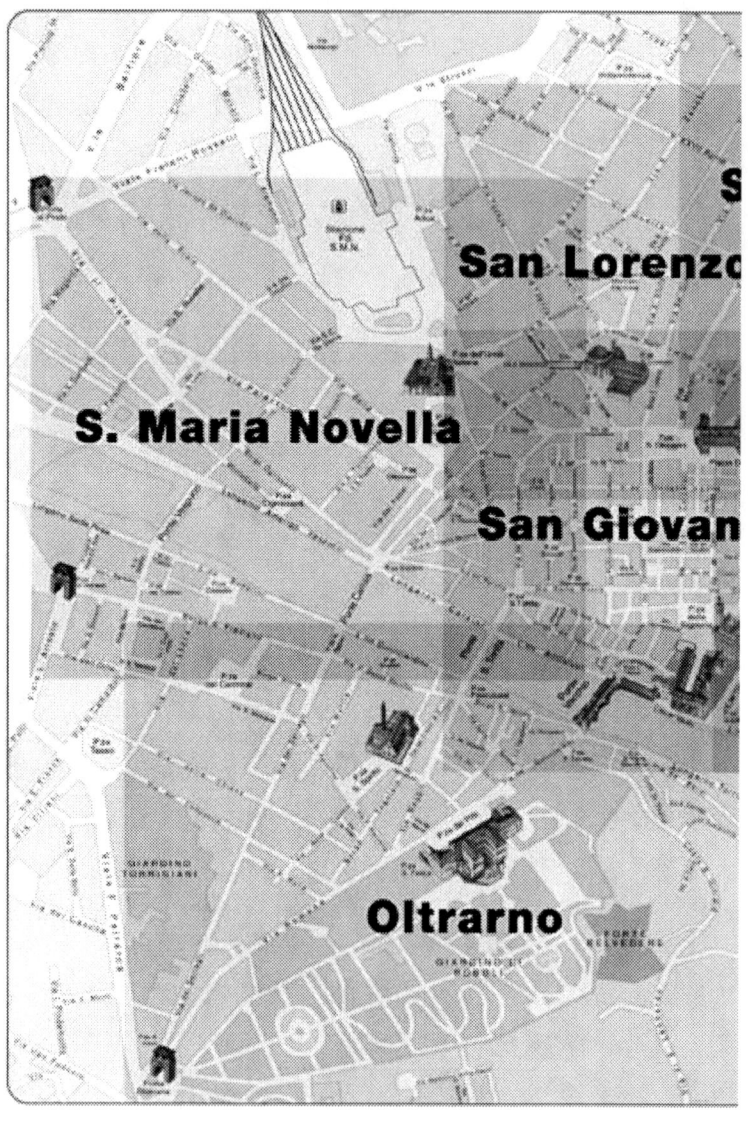

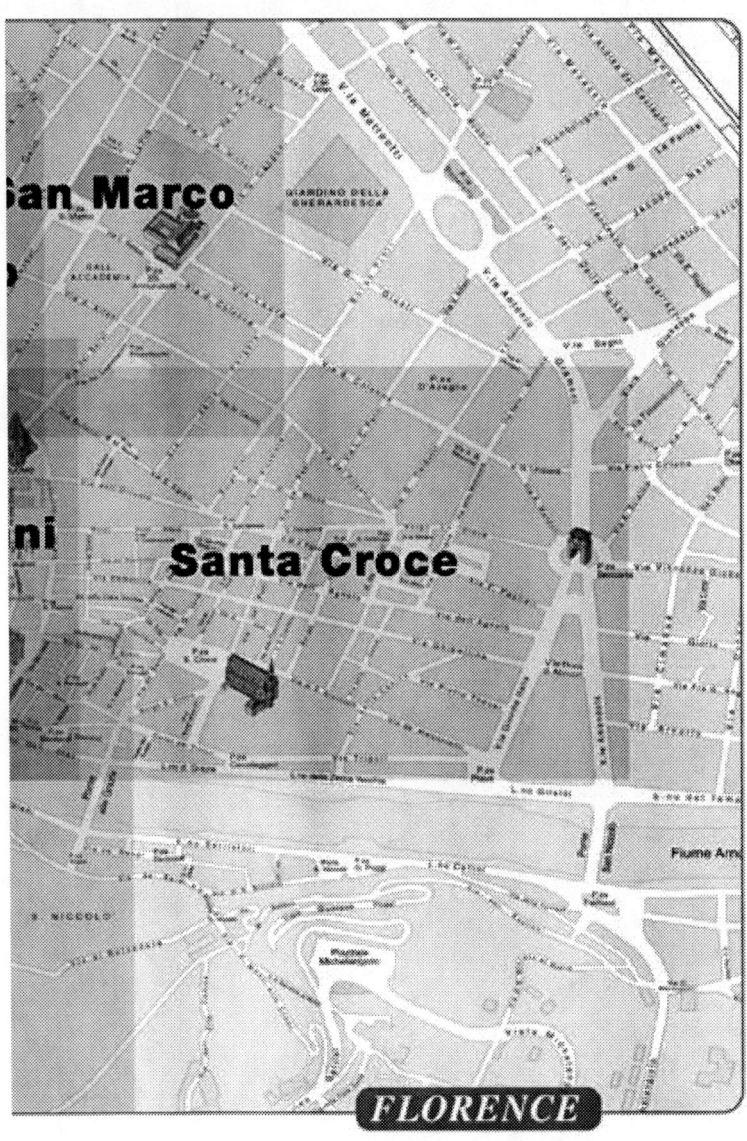

Introduction

Florence is a medium-sized city with a population of almost 377,000, not counting the six million tourists that visit each year. One would hope to find in such a big tourist town many more services equipped for visitors, not to mention residents, with disabilities, especially since the Italian government passed important legislation on disability in 1989, predating the "Americans with Disabilities Act" by one year.

In France the oft-heard phrase is *c'est la vie*; in Italy it is *pazienza*. Patience is indeed needed to cope with the Italians' often more relaxed attitude towards things, including compliance with building codes and the removal of architectural barriers. But then patience is needed by just about everybody who lives in or visits Italy, a country where some buildings date back to the days of the Roman Empire and where it is not unusual to find families living in a Renaissance palace or a fourteenth-century walkup. Some of the bumpy, stone-paved, traffic-congested narrow streets in cities like Rome and Florence hail back to medieval times. Even "wider" streets built in the sixteenth century to accommodate a new form of transportation—the carriage— were planned without sidewalks. In situations like these, installing a proper sidewalk with curb cuts sometimes just isn't possible.

Fortunately, 2000 marked a Jubilee Year for the Roman Catholic Church, and in anticipation of the millions of visitors, the Italian government allotted a significant amount of money in various major Italian cities to restore ancient buildings and generally to improve viability. As a consequence, many of the sidewalks in the *centro storico* or historic center of Florence were rebuilt with smoother stones and curb cuts, and several major churches like Santa Croce and Santo Spirito were equipped with ramps. The year 2003 was designated by the European Union as the "Year for People with Disabilities." The Regione Toscana or regional government of Tuscany, of which Florence is the principal city, celebrated with a weeklong series of sports and theatrical events and conferences on subjects ranging from architectural barriers to tourism and job opportunities. Initiatives like these mark a start in the right direction for a city like Florence, founded in 59 BC, to catch up to the twenty-first century.

Despite important improvements, Florence and Italy, in general, still present significant barriers to people with disabilities. The scenarios are numerous. How many hotels display the international wheelchair sign to indicate accessibility when, indeed, the interior of the hotel is accessible, but since it is located on the second floor with three steps in front of an elevator which is too small to accommodate a wheelchair, you can't get there. Imagine having lunch in an outdoor café in Piazza della Repubblica, soaking up the warm September sun, where do you find an accessible restroom? Where do you eat in a country whose main staples are bread, pizza, and pasta if you have an intolerance to wheat gluten? In which museums can you touch a Renaissance sculpture if you are visually impaired? Reading *The Accessible Guide to Florence* will answer these questions and, hopefully, many more.

This book does not pretend to be a complete guidebook to Florence. For a serious guide giving detailed historical and artistic descriptions, the best remain Eve Borsook's somewhat outdated but still valid *The Companion Guide to Florence* and Alta Macadam's *Florence,* part of the famous Blue Guide series. By far the most exhaustive guide to the city is the excellent *Firenze e Provincia* (in Italian only) published by the Italian Touring Club.

The Accessible Guide to Florence, instead, like many pocket guides, gives a briefer description of each monument, but one which still allows the reader to enjoy and understand enough without necessarily needing to bring along another guidebook. The chapters giving information on the monuments are organized according to geographical districts, and each is accompanied by a map for easier orientation. An accessibility "checklist" indicates the wheelchair-accessible banks, Internet points, pharmacies, restaurants, and restrooms in the neighborhood. General historical/artistic descriptions of each monument are followed by a detailed description of the monument's accessibility. There are chapters giving information on transportation, accommodations, places to eat, practical tips, and a brief history of the city. A guide explaining the mysteries of the metric system and a glossary with some useful phrases concerning accessibility are also included.

This guide is written primarily for slow walkers and wheelchair or scooter users, although some information has also been included for people with visual impairments, and a list of restaurants serving gluten-free meals is found in the chapter on "Places to Eat." Rather than creating a criteria for specific levels of accessibility, detailed descriptions, intended to allow each reader to judge independently whether a specific place will be in his case, or in her case, accessible, have been provided instead. However, as a general rule, any entrance with more than the 2.5-centimeter or 1-inch threshold lip allowed by Italian law has been defined as "accessible with assistance."

Two other important things should also be pointed out to readers consulting this book. Firstly, in general, platform lifts and stair lifts tend to be smaller and to have less weight capacity than their counterparts in the United States. Whenever possible, the exact dimensions and capacity of these lifts has been specified. Secondly, the majority of the streets and sidewalks in historic Florence are paved in stone and not covered with asphalt, which makes their surfaces highly unpredictable. Stable, firm, and slip-resistant accessible routes are difficult to come by, and one should always exert caution even in those areas which may be indicated as "accessible." Having said this, however, one can't fail to mention the exception to the rule since wheelchairs have been seen on the terrace of the Porcelain Museum and even heading up the steepest slopes of the Boboli Gardens.

While *The Accessible Guide to Florence* does not promise to become the "be all and end all" to everyone's needs, it is a first attempt to give visitors to Florence the tools for an honest assessment of what they can do and what they can see in this wonderful city.

History in a Nutshell

The Roman Settlement

It may be hard to imagine that Florence, so often labeled as the cradle of the Renaissance, has been around a lot longer; to be precise, for over two thousand years. A Roman colony was founded on the north bank of the Arno River during the reign of Julius Caesar, perhaps as early as 59 BC. Memories of the Roman settlement still remain in the names and configurations of some of the streets. The neat grid pattern in the heart of Florence's historic center between Via Tornabuoni, Piazza del Duomo, Via Proconsolo, and Piazza della Signoria defines the original layout of the fortified Roman town. Via delle Terme recalls the location of the Roman baths; Via del Campidoglio, where the main temple to Jupiter, Juno, and Minerva stood. The curving streets—Via Torta and Via de' Bentaccordi, together with Piazza de' Peruzzi near Piazza Santa Croce—follow the perimeter of the Roman amphitheatre. In the basement of the Cinema Gambrinus near Piazza della Repubblica, once heart of the Roman forum, you can still see some Roman foundations. The Roman colony, however, was not the earliest important settlement in the area. Up on the hills to the north an Etruscan city, now called Fiesole, overlooked the river valley and was considered around the sixth century BC to be one of the most important cities in northern Etruria. Later absorbed into the Roman Empire, during the Middle Ages Fiesole remained independent until conquered by Florence in the twelfth century.

Middle Ages

With the fall of the Western Roman Empire in 476, Florence, like the rest of Italy, was overrun by marauding barbarian tribes. The Dark Ages witnessed Goths and Byzantines struggling to gain control of the tiny settlement strategically located on the banks of the navigable Arno and near the foothills of the Apennine mountains with their important passes leading to the north. At the end of the sixth century, Florence fell under Lombard rule. Later, with the crowning of Charlemagne as Holy Roman Emperor in 800, she was tossed into the hands of the Carolingians. While much of the country officially came under Carolingian dominion, real control lay in the hands of the local feudal lords. In subsequent centuries, strong loyalties developed, and interests were split along a very clear line dividing those who were loyal to the pope in Rome from those who were loyal to the German kings. By the thirteenth century this division had created two strong political factions in Italy: the Guelphs and the Ghibellines. The ultimate split was already evident in the important and powerful figure of Matilda, countess of Tuscany, whose loyalty to the pope and desire to rid the peninsula of German rule led her to encourage the self-government of important walled cities like Florence. After Matilda's death in 1115, Florence gained the status of independent city state or *comune*.

During the twelfth and thirteen centuries, Florence witnessed a spurt of economic and demographic growth. Much of the city's good fortune was due to the development of the textile industry with a particular emphasis on the production of wool, the importance of which lasted up until the sixteenth century. Banking and the production of silk became other important activities, and by the early thirteenth century, Florence's influential business community was organized into powerful guilds. Florence's economic growth attracted outsiders to come and gain their fortune in the prosperous city, among them were the Medici who immigrated to town from an area north of Florence called the Mugello in the early twelfth century.

By 1200 the population of Florence had grown to fifty thousand; in 1280 there were eighty thousand people living in the city and probably one hundred thousand by 1300. At the time London's population numbered fifty thousand; Paris had two hundred thousand inhabitants, and Florence ranked together with her as one of the five largest cities in Europe. In 1284 Arnolfo di Cambio directed the construction of a new ring of city walls to accommodate the ever-growing population. The walls were finished in 1333, but in 1348 the plague, known as the Black Death, devastated the city, cutting its numbers in half. Small farms with open fields and orchards were to abound in large areas within the new walls well into the nineteenth century when the former population finally managed to catch up with itself.

The Medici

Guelph and Ghibelline differences came to a head with the defeat of the Ghibellines in 1267, and within a small group of Florentine merchants and Guelph sympathizers, the Medici began to make their way towards political and economic power. Except for a brief interim between 1494 and 1530, Florence was ruled, either behind the scenes or officially, by the Medici family for almost three hundred years between 1434 and 1743.

Giovanni di Bicci de' Medici (1360-1429) paved the way for his descendents by building an influential banking empire, whose clients also included the pope. His oldest son **Cosimo il Vecchio** (the Elder) (1389-1464), also known as Cosimo il Pater Patriae (Father of his Country), managed to rule Florence informally through the influence of his economic position while never holding an important seat within the government. Patron of important architectural projects such as the Convent of San Marco and his own family palace near San Lorenzo, friend of famous artists like Donatello, founder of an academy devoted to the study of Plato, he was a true "Renaissance man." His grandson **Lorenzo the Magnificent** (1449-1492) carried on the family's cultural traditions. A gifted poet and armchair architect, he also promoted the careers of aspiring young artists like Leonardo and Michelangelo.

Absolute Medici rule was not sealed in the fifteenth century with rival factions trying to seize their power. Cosimo had already been driven into exile in Venice before returning in 1434. Lorenzo the Magnificent nearly lost his life in 1478 in the Pazzi Conspiracy. His son, Piero, weak in character, was not able to sustain the brilliant reputation of his father and grandfather, and political ineptitude forced him to surrender the city to the French in 1494. Soon after, a republic was formed with the fanatic Dominican priest from San Marco, **Savonarola**, at its head. Urging the Florentines to throw their profane books, cosmetics, portraits of beautiful women, jewelry, playing cards, and dice into "vanity bonfires," he led them to believe that their true leader was God. The Florentines, however, had little patience for this regime of austerity, and in 1498, Savonarola's career was cut short when he was burned at the stake as a heretic in front of Palazzo Vecchio. The Republic was to linger on for another fourteen years until Lorenzo the Magnificent's younger son, Giovanni, rode into Florence with the support of the pope to reclaim his inheritance and to restore Medici rule. Three years later, Giovanni returned as **Pope Leo X** (1475-1521), one of the most brilliant Renaissance papal patrons of art whose fine portrait by Raphael today hangs in the Uffizi.

When Rome was sacked by the troops of the emperor Charles V in 1527, anti-Medicean factions seized the opportunity to force the Medici once again into exile. Thanks to an alliance between Charles and another famous Medici **Pope Clement VII** (1478-1534), who, only three years earlier, had been driven out of Rome by the emperor, the Medici were allowed to return in 1530. **Alessandro de' Medici** (1511-1537), reputedly Pope Clement's illegitimate son, was nominated duke, and a marriage was arranged with the emperor's daughter to solidify the new alliance. When the unpopular Alessandro was assassinated in 1537, supporters of the Republic saw their last chance to regain hold of the government slip away as power passed to **Cosimo I** (1519-74), descendant of a younger son of Giovanni di Bicci. When Cosimo I was granted the title of grand duke of Tuscany in 1569, the Medici dynasty was secured as power from then on was passed from father to son. Both successors of Cosimo I, his first son **Francesco I** (1541-87) to be succeeded by **Ferdinando I** (1549-1609), were important Medici rulers and patrons of art during the late Renaissance.

Transition

With the death of the last male Medici in 1737, rule was granted by treaty to the French House of Lorraine. The illuminated reign of the Lorraine grand duke **Pietro Leopoldo** (1765-1790) was outstanding for its reforms in agriculture, education, and health, and under his rule, Florence witnessed the abolition of the death penalty, the introduction of the Gregorian calendar, the creation of a chamber of commerce to replace the old guild system, and the opening of new schools for the education of the poor. With the rise of Napoleon, the Lorraine were expelled in 1799. Florence then became part of the Kingdom of Etruria and, for a short period, was ruled by Napoleon's sister, Elisa Bonaparte Baciocchi, between 1809 and 1814. The Lorraine were then reinstated and, except for a brief interim, continued to govern until a few months before Florence became part of the newly unified Kingdom of Italy in 1860. From 1865 to 1870 Florence served as capital city of the new country and was home to her first king, **Victor Emmanuel II** (1820-1878).

Florence in the Twentieth Century

Several tragic events were to mark Florentine history in the twentieth century. During the Second World War many of the transportable art treasures were taken into the Tuscan countryside for safekeeping, but not everything could be saved. In 1944, as they retreated from allied advance, the Germans destroyed all the city's historic bridges, except for the Ponte Vecchio. To save it, the medieval streets on both sides of the bridge were reduced to rubble, and an astute eye will see today that most of the buildings at the lower part of Via Por San Maria and Via Guicciardini on either side of the bridge are modern constructions. On November 4, 1966, another tragedy struck the city. In the dark of the night, the waters of the Arno rose to six meters (19 ½ feet) above street level. Mixed with mud blacked by fuel oil used for heating, the raging waters spread throughout the city. Fourteen thousand people were left homeless, thousands of shops were put out of business, and countless works of art and historical monuments were damaged or destroyed as so eloquently testified by one of the famous survivors: Cimabue's *Crucifixion* at Santa Croce. Another blow to the city's cultural heritage came in 1993 when a Mafia bomb exploded behind the Uffizi, killing five people, destroying the historic library of the eighteenth-century Accademia dei Georgofili, and causing serious damage to the Uffizi and Vasari's corridor.

The Renaissance: Art, Music, Literature, and Science

Throughout her long history, the highlight of Florence's cultural achievement remains her contribution to the Renaissance. With the revival of ancient Greek and Roman art and language, the Age of the Renaissance sparked off a new interest in classical studies in disciplines ranging from philosophy to architecture, mathematics to painting. Renaissance men like Cosimo de'Medici sent their agents throughout Europe and into the Near East seeking classical texts for their private libraries in monasteries which for centuries had preserved the ancient writings. The humanist **Marsilio Ficino** (1433-1499) translated all of Plato's works into Latin and was director of the Platonic Academy, of which Cosimo de'Medici was also a founding member, devoted to the study of the Greek philosopher. **Donatello** (1386-1466), the sculptor, created new marvelously naturalistic statues, so lifelike that he once commanded one to speak. **Brunelleschi** (1377-1446), the architect, brought a new sense of order and harmony of proportion to Florentine architecture. Both their achievements were based on the direct observation of classical art as recounted by **Giorgio Vasari** (1511-

1574) in his famous *Lives of the Artists* who described a trip to Rome made together by the two artists in the early fifteenth century to study the ancient ruins practically "neglecting to sleep and eat . . . and leaving nothing unvisited . . ." so great was their fascination with the ancient city. **Masaccio** (1401-1428) was the third link in bringing about similar revolutions in painting by successfully creating realistic representations of space, volume, structure, and three-dimensional form on a two-dimensional painted surface. In mentioning the Florentine Renaissance, one cannot overlook the importance of other Florentine artists: the sculptor **Ghiberti** (1378-1455), creator of the Baptistery gilded bronze doors known as the *Gates of Paradise*; the painters **Fra Angelico** (1400-1455) who decorated the Convent of San Marco and **Botticelli** (1455-1510) whose most famous paintings, the *Birth of Venus* and *Primavera*, were commissioned by members of the Medici family. **Leonardo da Vinci** (1452-1519) and **Michelangelo** (1474-1564) both lived and worked in Florence for part of their outstanding careers. In speaking of Florence's contribution, one cannot fail to mention **Dante Alighieri** (1265-1321), author of the *Divine Comedy*, the first important work of literature to be written in vernacular Italian, the poet **Petrarch** (1304-1374), and **Boccaccio** (1312-1375), author of the *Decameron*. **Galileo** (1564-1642), one of the fathers of modern science, lived and died in Florence where major contributions in the field of music were also made. The pianoforte was invented in 1711 by **Bartolomeo Cristofori** (1655-1731), and lyric opera made its first appearance in 1600 in the performance of Iacopo Peri's "Euridice" during festivities held to honor the marriage of Grand Duke Cosimo I's granddaughter Maria to King Henry IV of France.

LEGEND

 Monument

 Accommodation

 Place to eat

 Monument with accessible restroom

 Accommodation with public accessible WC

 Place to eat with accessible restroom

 Accessible restroom

 Tourist Information

 Taxi

 Cinema

 Theater

 Box Office

 Bank

 Exchange Bureau

 ATM

 Parking with at least one designated space

 Internet Point

 Travel Agency

 Post Office

 Hospital

 Pharmacy

San Giovanni

From the Duomo to Palazzo Vecchio, Piazza della Repubblica, and Via Tornabuoni

The district of San Giovanni is named after St. John the Baptist, Florence's patron saint, whose name is appropriately bestowed on the Baptistery located in front of the cathedral popularly known as the **Duomo**. From Piazza del Duomo, Via Calzaiuoli leads past the guild Church of **Orsanmichele** to the city government palace **Palazzo Vecchio** in Piazza della Signoria, thus connecting the two poles representing Florence's religious and political power. Statues and fountains decorate the Signoria Square: Duke Cosimo I sits astride a great bronze horse, much like the statue of Marcus Aurelius on Rome's Capitoline Hill, proving that the Medici never tired of drawing parallels between themselves and great figures from Roman history. The Neptune fountain alludes to Medici naval pursuits in the Mediterranean, while a replica of David, placed in its original position next to the front door of the government palace, is a civic symbol of Florentine liberty.

The **Loggia dei Lanzi,** a fourteenth-century portico built for government ceremonies and decorated with statuary including Benvenuto Cellini's bronze *Perseus*, faces the square. Around the corner the **Uffizi** or "offices," now a world-famous art museum, were built in the sixteenth century by order of Duke Cosimo I as a government office building. Nearby the duke ordered the construction of a new market loggia, the

Mercato Nuovo, for the sale of precious objects and cloth. Today the market, popularly known as the Loggia del Porcellino, sells leather goods and tourist souvenirs. The street of Por Santa Maria leads past the market to the **Ponte Vecchio,** the oldest bridge across the Arno, whose gold shops replaced unsightly butcher stalls when the Medici ordered a raised corridor to be built over the bridge in 1565, both to commemorate the wedding of Cosimo's eldest son, Francesco, and to connect the two family palaces on opposite sides of the river, the suburban Palazzo Pitti to the town residence in Palazzo Vecchio.

In **Piazza della Repubblica,** a column marks the point where the two main streets, the north-south cardo and the east-west decumanus, met at the center of the old Roman town settlement. Now nineteenth-century palaces, porticoes, and lively cafés line the edges of this relatively "new" piazza, once the site of the old Roman forum and later of a busy Renaissance marketplace. To the west, **Via Tornabuoni,** with its elegant shops, leads past the **Church of Santa Trinita** to the **Santa Trinita Bridge** built by Ammannati, possibly after a design by Michelangelo, and decorated with marble statues of the four seasons in occasion of a seventeenth-century Medici wedding. Across the bridge lies the neighborhood known as the Oltrarno.

Mobility

Getting There

The following bus routes pass through the neighborhood of San Giovanni:

Wheelchair-accessible Bus 23 (direction "Sorgane") leaves the west side of the RR station, making stops near Piazza del Duomo, in Via del Proconsolo (two blocks from the entrance to the Bargello Museum), and behind Palazzo Vecchio (also good for the Uffizi and the Museo di Storia della Scienza) before crossing the river.

The reverse route (direction "Zona Industriale") from Piazza Ferrucci passes by Santa Croce and the Duomo, on the way back to the station.

Electric Bus A (direction "Beccaria") leaves the RR station outside "Departures" making stops in Piazza Santa Maria Novella, in Piazza Ognissanti, in Via del Parione near the Church of Santa Trinita, in Via Tornabuoni, near the Duomo in Via dei Pecori, in Piazza della Repubblica, Orsanmichele, Piazza Ciompi, and Piazza Beccaria. The reverse direction ("Stazione") leaves from Piazza Beccaria passing by Piazza San Pier Maggiore, Via della Condotta, Piazza della Repubblica, Palazzo Strozzi, Piazza Santa Maria Novella, ending its route at the station.

Electric Bus B (direction "Piave") makes stops east of Ponte della Vittoria near the Cascine Park, in Via Curtatone near the American Consulate, in Lungarno Vespucci near the Church of the Ognissanti and Ghirlandaio's *Last Supper,* in Via del Parione (Church of Santa Trinita), near the Ponte Vecchio, the Uffizi and Museo di Storia della Scienza. The reverse direction ("Fonderia") makes the following stops: "Biblioteca Nazionale" (for Santa Croce), "Loggia del Grano" (Museo di Storia e della Scienza), "Vacchereccia" (Piazza della Signoria), "SS Apostoli," Piazza Santa Trinita, Piazza Goldoni, and Ponte alla Carraia.

Getting Around

Getting around is relatively easy in this neighborhood which is the heart of the *centro storico.* Much of the area between the Piazza del Duomo and the river is closed to regular traffic, and many sidewalks have recently been rebuilt with curb cuts. Even so, this guidebook would like to emphasize that the entire *centro storico,* including the district of San Giovanni, is, by nature of the stone used to pave streets and sidewalks, unpredictable in terms of its accessibility and that one should always use extreme caution even in those areas which are indicated as accessible without assistance in the "Map on Urban Accessibility" published by the city of Florence.

While Via Calzaiuoli (the main route between Piazza del Duomo and Piazza della Signoria), Piazza del Duomo, Piazza della Signoria, and Piazza della Repubblica are pedestrian zones, be on the lookout for bicycles, taxis, electric buses, and horse-drawn carriages.

Most of the stores under the portico in Piazza della Repubblica are accessible to wheelchairs.

Taxi stands are located in Piazza Santa Trinita, Piazza della Repubblica, Via de'Pecori near Piazza San Giovanni, and behind the Duomo.

Driving is restricted, and designated parking is especially difficult to find in this area of town which is part of the ZTL (Limited Traffic Zone). To enter with a car, you will need special permission (see chapter on "Transportation" under "Driving Around"). There is one designated parking space in Piazza Santa Trinita; another is on the east side of Via de'Vecchietti near Via dei Cerretani, the main street between the Duomo and the RR station. By tacit agreement, disability parking permit holders who have received permission to enter the ZTL are allowed to park inside the chained-off area behind the Duomo, in Piazza della Signoria on the north side of Palazzo Vecchio opposite the wheelchair-accessible entrance, and on the north and south edges of Piazza della Repubblica, even though these parking spaces are not marked. Several other unmarked places are mentioned in the guide *The Florence Experience*.

What the Neighborhood Has to Offer

Outdoor cafés in Piazza della Repubblica and Piazza della Signoria, two major department stores—La Rinascente and

Coin, a host of shoe and leather shops, clothing boutiques, and the main post office are found in the neighborhood of San Giovanni. Try some ice cream at **Perchè No** (why not?) in Via dei Tavolini (*low step at entrance: 8 centimeters [3 ¹/₈ inches]*), a club sandwich at **Gilli** in Piazza della Repubblica, a summertime *granita di café con panna* (ice coffee topped with whipped cream), or a wintertime *cioccolata calda con panna* (hot chocolate with whipped cream) at **Rivoire** in Piazza della Signoria. Behind the Baptistery, you'll find **Scudieri**, a well-known bar/pasticceria in Piazza San Giovanni, with level entrance and outside seating. **Coin** in Via Calzaioli and **La Rinascente** in Piazza della Repubblica are two chain department stores with wheelchair-accessible restrooms, and at La Rinascente, there is an accessible, top-floor café on an open loggia overlooking the piazza with a spectacular close-up view of Brunelleschi's cupola. **La Cantinetta dei Verrazzano** in Via de'Tavolini is a good place for a morning coffee and pastry or lunchtime pasta and a glass of wine. If you're on the run and don't mind eating on the sidewalk, try **I Fratellini** in Via dei Cimatori, 38/r, an over-the-counter food stall selling wine and *panini* or the tripe vendor in Piazza del Mercato Nuovo. For a proper sit-down meal, the **Ristorante/ Pizzeria Il Bargello** in Piazza della Signoria also has outside seating, or there is the newly opened restaurant **Al Lume di Candela** in Via delle Terme. (*One step at entrance. Ring bell for assistance in entering.*) If you are fond of truffles, **Procacci** in Via Tornabuoni, 64/r, has been serving its mouth-watering truffle sandwiches since 1885. The city's **main post office** is in Via Pellicceria, just off Piazza della Repubblica. Open Monday-Friday, 8:15-19:00, and on Saturday, 8:15-12:30. There are six steps at main entrance. The wheelchair-accessible entrance is located at the rear of the post office in Via de'Sassetti, 2. (*Ring bell to open the gate and follow the ramp to the left of the courtyard into the main hall.*)

Accessibility Checklist

The following list contains places which are accessible to people in wheelchairs.

Accommodations

- Hotel Benivieni
- Hotel dell'Orafo
- Hotel Pierre
- Hotel Porta Rossa
- Hotel Savoy

Places to Eat

Piazza del Duomo

- Caffè Duomo
- Scudieri
  No accessible restroom.

Piazza della Repubblica

- Gilli
  Outside seating. Step at entrance to inside seating: 7 centimeters (2 ¾ inches). No accessible restroom.
- Giubbe Rosse
  Outside seating. Step at entrance. No accessible restroom.
- Hotel Savoy
  The café/bar has both outside and inside seating. Restaurant inside. Accessible restroom.
- Paszkowski
  Ramped entrance to outside seating area is from the piazza. Step at the entrance to inside seating. No accessible restroom.
- Terrace Café at La Rinascente
  Take the main elevator to the top floor, then transfer to a

smaller elevator, located on the west side of the store, which takes you up to the roof. The button must be kept pushed in for the elevator to move (elevator door: 89 centimeters [35 inches] wide; cabin depth: 115 centimeters [45 ¼ inches]). Table and chairs, placed too close to the elevator door, make exiting sometimes difficult at the lower bar level. No difficulty is encountered in exiting for the café on the roof. An accessible restroom is located on the top floor of the store (southeast corner). (See chapter on "Practical Tips and Useful Information" under "Restrooms" for description.)

Piazza della Signoria

The outside seating of most cafés and trattorie around the piazza can be accessed from the sidewalk in a wheelchair; the places mentioned below also have accessible restrooms.

- Hot Pot
- Ristorante/Pizzeria Il Bargello
- Uffizi
  The café/bar is located inside the gallery on the top floor.

Others

- Al Lume di Candela
  Step at entrance. Ring bell for assistance.
- Da Pennello
  Low step (7 centimeters [2 ¾ inches]) at entrance. Ramp inside front door. No accessible restroom.
- I Buongustai
  Narrow ramped entrance. Recommended for smaller manual chairs.
- La Cantinetta dei Verrazzano
- Robiglio

Outside and inside seating. One step at entrance to bar. Ring bell for assistance. There is a short ramp at a side door to the lunchroom and to the accessible restroom which is located through the big arched doorway to the left of the entrance to the bar in Via de' Tosinghi.

- Uffizi Center
  Wheelchair-accessible entrance is presently from Via del Castello d'Altafronte, the street to the left of the main entrance in Via de' Neri.

Accessible Restrooms

Piazza del Duomo

- Museo dell'Opera del Duomo
- Caffè Duomo

Piazza della Repubblica

- La Rinascente Department Store
- Hotel Savoy

Piazza della Signoria

- Hot Pot
- Palazzo Vecchio
- Ristorante/Pizzeria Il Bargello
- Uffizi

Others

- Al Lume di Candela
- Coin Department Store
- I Buongustai
- La Cantinetta dei Verrazzano
- Museo di Storia della Scienza
- Palazzo Strozzi

- Robiglio
- Uffizi Center

Miscellaneous

Lowered ATM machines

- Palazzo Vecchio
  Located to the right inside the wheelchair-accessible entrance. The entrance is open between 8:00 and 19:00.
- Banca Toscana
  Piazza della Signoria 22/r
  Requires a reach for a person under five feet five inches.
- Banca San Paolo
  Piazza della Repubblica, 4 at the corner of Via Pellicceria
  Requires a reach for a person under five feet five inches.
- Banca Popolare di Novara
  Via Pellicceria, 34/r
  Requires a reach for a person under five feet five inches.

Banks

Piazza della Signoria

- Banca Toscana
  Piazza della Signoria 22/r
  Both the entrance to the bank and the ATM machine outside are accessible to wheelchairs.

Piazza della Repubblica

- Banca Nazionale del Lavoro
  Piazza della Repubblica, 21/r (under the left portico)
  There are two successive, automatic doors at the entrance. The first door opens, allowing you to enter a space sufficiently

large enough for a wheelchair. Once this door closes, the second door opens. Bell at entrance for assistance in entering, if needed.

- Cassa di Risparmio, Agenzia 16
Via degli Speziali, 18/r (across from La Rinascente Department Store)
The wheelchair-accessible entrance, which doubles as a safety exit, is normally kept locked. There is a bell to ring for assistance.

- Rolo Banca 1473
Via Brunelleschi, 11 (at the north end of the portico)
Heavy, self-operating glass entrance doors. No bell.

Exchange Bureau

- Cambio Exchange
Porta Santa Maria, 3/r (just off the Ponte Vecchio)
The window has a high counter and is open to the street. There is a rise, about 4 centimeters (1 ½ inches), at the threshold.

Internet Points

- Internet Service
Piazza della Signoria, 37/r
The wheelchair-accessible entrance is around the corner in Via dei Magazzini, 1. Since this door is normally closed, you will have to request that it be opened.

Pharmacies

- Farmacia all'Insegna del Moro
Piazza di San Giovanni, 20/r

Tel: 055 211 343
Slight lip at entrance.

- Farmacia Internazionale
  Piazza della Repubblica, 23/r
  Tel: 055 210 713

- Farmacia Molteni
  Via Calzaiuoli, 7/r
  Tel: 055 215 472
  There is a 4-centimeter (1 ½-inch) threshold lip at entrance. The pharmacy is open twenty-four hours.

- Farmacia del Corso
  Via del Corso, 13/r
  Tel: 055 210 217

Travel Agencies

- Pellegrinaggi Viaggi
  Piazza San Giovanni, 4
  Tel: 055 216 003

San Giovanni

Monuments

1. Baptistery
2. Duomo and Bell Tower
3. Loggia del Bigallo
4. Museo dell'Opera del Duomo
5. Church of Orsanmichele
6. Badia Fiorentina
7. Casa di Dante
8. Palazzo Vecchio
9. Uffizi
10. Mercato Nuovo
11. Museo di Storia della Scienza
12. Museo Ferragamo
13. Palazzo Davanzati
14. Palazzo Strozzi
15. Church of SS. Apostoli
16. Church of Santa Trinita

Places to Eat

1. Caffè Duomo
2. Scudieri
3. Terrace Café and Box Office
4. Hot Pot
5. Ristorante/Pizzeria Bargello
6. Rivoire
7. Al Lume di Candela
8. Trattoria da Pennello
9. I Buongustai
10. La Cantinetta dei Verrazzano
11. Robiglio
12. Antico Fattore
13. Café Uffizi
14. Uffizi Center

Accommodations

1. Hotel Benivieni
2. Hotel dell'Orafo
3. Hotel Pierre
4. Hotel Porta Rossa
5. Hotel Savoy

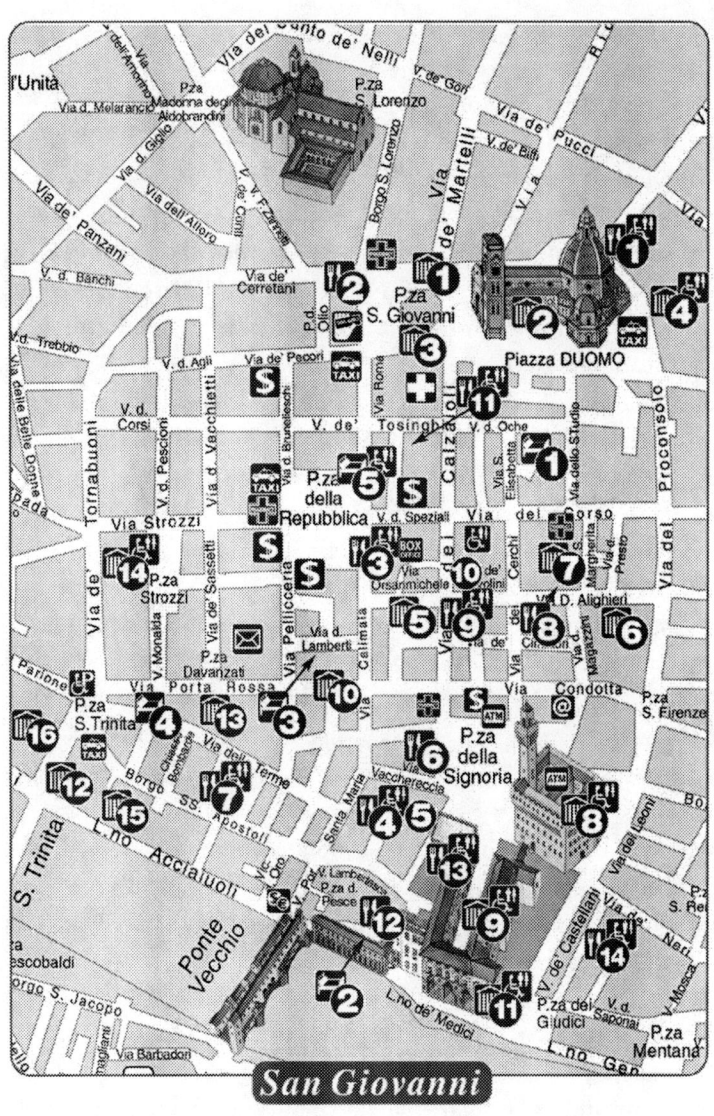

San Giovanni

What to See

Around the Duomo

Baptistery (accessible with assistance)
Piazza del Duomo
Tel: Opera del Duomo 055 230 2885
Open: Monday-Saturday, 12:00-19:00; Sunday, 8:30-14:00
Admission: €3,00

Description: Tradition has it that a temple dedicated to Mars once stood on this site, but some mosaic pavement, brought to light during excavations, indicates that the precedent building was not a Roman temple, but probably a bakery. The highly classical window frames and orders decorating the facade led Renaissance architects like Leon Battista Alberti to believe the Baptistery really was Roman even though its construction was not begun until the mid-eleventh century. There was no penny pinching when it came to decorating this very important monument dedicated to Florence's patron, San Giovanni. Of the three sets of magnificent bronze doors on the exterior, the most famous were the gilded doors facing the Duomo designed by Lorenzo Ghiberti (1425-1452). Nicknamed by Michelangelo, the *Gates of Paradise*, the original panels are now on view in the courtyard of the Museo dell'Opera del Duomo. In the thirteenth century specialists were called from Venice and Byzantium to decorate the interior of the octagonal dome in mosaic with stories depicting the Creation, Joseph and his brothers, John the Baptist, and the Virgin and Christ, together with the Last Judgment and a terrifying scene of the damned in hell.

Accessibility: There is one step at the entrance threshold (12 centimeters [4 ¾ inches] outer side; 6 centimeters [2 ³/₈ inches] on the inside). The guard will dismantle the gate at the ticket booth to allow for the passage of a wheelchair. A small ramp leads from the ticket booth area to floor level; inside there are no obstacles.

To exit, leave by the entrance door since the step at the exit door threshold is higher. Seating is available.

Comments: A free (but not always accurate) pamphlet in English, describing the history of the Baptistery and cathedral, is available from a little stand located inside the entrance door on the left.

Campanile di Giotto (not accessible)
Piazza San Giovanni
Tel: 055 230 2885
Open: 8:30-19:30
Admission: €6,00

Description: Designed by Giotto in 1334, work was continued on the bell tower by Andrea Pisano and completed by Francesco Talenti in 1359. The statues of prophets and patriarchs that once decorated its facade, together with the bas reliefs, some designed by Giotto, have been replaced by copies. The originals can be seen in the Museo dell'Opera del Duomo, including Donatello's *Zuccone*, the statue that appeared so real to the artist that, as legend has it, he commanded it to speak.

Accessibility: There are about four hundred steps to the top of the tower. No elevator.

Duomo (Santa Maria del Fiore) (accessible with assistance)
Piazza del Duomo
Tel: Opera del Duomo 055 230 2885
Home Page: *www.operaduomo.firenze.it*
Open: Weekdays, 10:00-17:00, except Thursday, 10:00-15:30; Saturday, 10:00-16:45, except first Saturday of the month, 10:00-15:30; Sundays and holidays, 13:30-16:45
Admission: Free
Other: Mass is held in English at 17:00 on Saturday evenings, except for the first Saturday of the month when it is held at the Misericordia located across from Giotto's bell tower. *(There are*

four steps at the entrance to the Misericordia Chapel, but the attendants on duty will assist carrying wheelchairs up the steps.)

Description: The Duomo or cathedral was begun around 1296 after a design by Arnolfo di Cambio, architect of Palazzo Vecchio, Santa Croce, and the last ring of city walls. Construction on the project, which turned out to be the fourth-largest church in the world, dragged on for over 150 years. Its double shell dome, designed in 1425 by the architect Filippo Brunelleschi, was one of the engineering feats of the Renaissance. Officially the cathedral is known as Santa Maria del Fiore, Saint Mary "of the Flower," alluding to Florence's symbol, the lily, but the name really harks back to pagan origins when the Roman settlement of "Fiorentia" was founded during the springtime festivities celebrating Flora, Roman goddess of flowers.

During the Renaissance and up until the latter nineteenth century, the Duomo's unfinished facade looked very much like that of nearby Church of San Lorenzo. The polychrome marble main facade seen today, like that of Santa Croce, is a neo-Gothic addition. Especially by comparison to its present colorful exterior, the interior of the Duomo appears strikingly solemn and bare. Much of the decorative trappings have been removed, partly due to changing taste, partly for reasons of conservation, to the Museo dell'Opera del Duomo, and a visit to this museum is a must in order to get a full idea of the past magnificence of Florence's cathedral.

Accessibility: The main entrance has six steps and no handrail. The wheelchair-accessible entrance (with threshold lip: 6 centimeters [2 ³/₈ inches]) is on the south side of the cathedral behind Giotto's bell tower. Inside the main door, there are wooden inner doors. The wider central door can be opened by the guard standing inside the entrance. The narrower side doors have a width of 77 centimeters (30 ¼ inches). The nave and presbytery are barrier free except for one step (up: 17 centimeters [6 ¾ inches]; down: 6 centimeters [2 ³/₈ inches]) to view through glass doors into the sacristy and fourteen steps leading down to the level of the bookstore and to the excavations of Santa Reparata, the old cathedral buried under the later construction. (Admission fee: €3,00) There are 463 steps up to the top of Brunelleschi's dome (admission fee).

Comments: Two wheelchairs are available at the main entrance for use of visitors. Free guided tours in English are offered.

Loggia del Bigallo (not accessible)
Piazza San Giovanni
Tel: 055 215 440
Open: 10:00-18:00 everyday, except Tuesday
Admission: €2,00

Description: The fourteenth-century *loggia* was originally built for the *Misericordia,* a religious society whose good deeds included accompanying the sick to hospitals and burying the dead. Today the *Misericordia* provides a medical and ambulance service with headquarters in the corner building opposite Giotto's bell tower. In the late fifteenth century, the *Misericordia* ceded the loggia to the *Compagnia di Santa Maria del Bigallo,* a charitable organization devoted to looking after lost and abandoned children. When found, the unfortunate children were first displayed from the porch, and if no one came forth to claim them, they were taken in by the *Compagnia.* Today the loggia and the Bigallo headquarters house a small museum containing a few fourteenth-century paintings and frescoes including the *Madonna of the Misericordia* with one of the oldest known painted scenes of Florence in the background.

Accessibility: Not accessible to wheelchairs. There are three steps at the entrance to this tiny museum consisting of three rooms. Once inside the museum, between the first and second rooms, there is a step down (17 centimeters [6 ¾ inches]) through a narrow door (65 centimeters [25 ⅝ inches] wide).

Museo dell'Opera del Duomo

Piazza Duomo, 9 (behind the Duomo)
Tel: 055 230 2885
Open: Monday-Saturday, 9:00-19:30; Sunday, 9:00-13:40
Admission: €6,00; credit cards are accepted for a minimum of €30,00

Description: Decorative objects from the Duomo's interior and its original medieval facade, from Giotto's bell tower and from the Baptistery, are now housed in the Museo dell'Opera del Duomo. Not to miss are the choir lofts by Donatello and Luca della Robbia, a haunting *Mary Magdalene* by Donatello, Ghiberti's original panels from the Baptistery *Gates of Paradise* doors, and a late *Pietà* by Michelangelo.

Accessibility: This newly renovated museum is almost entirely barrier free. The main entrance from the street into the ticket hall is wheelchair accessible. From the ticket hall, a guard will let you through the gate at the left of the turnstile for entrance into the galleries. An **accessible restroom** is located on the ground floor immediately inside this gate (WC has lateral transfer space and retractable grab bar on left; fixed grab bar on right wall; the metal pipe under the sink is not wrapped). A **second accessible larger restroom** is located upstairs on level 2 (WC has lateral transfer space and retractable grab bar on left; fixed grab bar on right wall).

Ground-floor rooms are all wheelchair accessible, but to reach the *Sala dei corali* and chapel (three steps up), you will have to backtrack. Leave the hall with the medieval sculpture from the Duomo facade and go through the vestibule into the atrium near the main stairs. Through a wooden door next to the medieval sculpture hall which you have just left is a self-operated platform lift.

Two **elevators** to the upper floors are located in the main courtyard. The elevator on the right is slightly larger and reaches all levels (door: 89 centimeters [35 inches]; cabin width: 144 centimeters [56 ¾ inches]; cabin length: 137 centimeters [54 inches]). Go to level 1 for Michelangelo's *Pietà*; level 2 for the accessible restroom; level 3 for the main exhibition rooms. All of the rooms on level 3 are fully accessible except for the rear part of the room containing Donatello's *Mary Magdalene* where there are five steps up to view the silver altar from the Baptistery. A ramp located in the room with the bell tower relief panels also connects level 3 to level 2. Level 4 contains only a few pieces of sculpture and fresco fragments.

Seating is available in the larger rooms. Guided touch tours are given by advance appointment only for visitors with visual impairments (for further information see "Museums, Music, Movies, and Sports").

Comments: The museum is air-conditioned and well organized, with explanatory panels in English and Italian and a very helpful staff. Free guided tours are given in English on the hour between 13:00 and 16:00 (1:00 p.m. to 4:00 p.m.).

In Via Calzaiuoli

Orsanmichele (interior not accessible)
Via Calzaiuoli near Piazza della Signoria. Entrance is from Via Arte della Lana.
Tel: 055 284 944
Open: Temporarily closed but open on rare occasions for concerts
Admission: Tickets must be purchased for concerts.

Description: In 1290, a loggia designed by Arnolfo di Cambio, architect of the Duomo, was built as a grain market in the garden or *orto* of San Michele. Destroyed by fire in the early fourteenth century, the loggia was rebuilt and, in following years, modified to include a granary upstairs and a ground-floor oratory. Later, when the arches were walled in, Orsanmichele became a church, and much of its decoration was delegated to the guilds of Florence. The interior of the church is decorated with images of their patron saints painted on the pillars, and a lavish marble tabernacle was designed by Orcagna to house a miraculous image of the Virgin. The decision to fill the niches of the exterior facade with monumental sculpture resulted in the brilliant display of some of the most remarkable talent of Renaissance Florence. Huge bronze statues once occupied the three niches on the Via Calzaiuoli facade: Ghiberti's *St. John the Baptist,* Verrocchio's *Doubting Thomas,* and Giambologna's *St. Luke.* Around the corner, Donatello's intensely psychological and realistic *St. George* was commissioned by the Guild of the Armorers. Next to it are the Mason's and Carpenter's Guild statues by Nanni di Banco of the *Quattro Coronati,* four Early Christian saints who were martyred for their refusal to make a pagan image of the emperor. Today replicas are gradually being put in place of the statues. Donatello's marble *St. George* is now in the Bargello while most of the other originals are on display upstairs in the Orsanmichele Museum (not accessible).

Accessibility: The normal entrance in Via Arte della Lana involves two steps and a sharp turn to the right through the inner door. The museum (not accessible) is located on the upper floors above the church. There is no elevator. Entrance to the museum is opposite the church in Via Arte della Lana.

Around Piazza della Signoria

Badia Fiorentina (not accessible)
Via Dante Alighieri
Tel: 055 283 451
Open: Monday only, 15:00-18:00
Admission: Free

Description: This Benedictine monastery, founded in AD 978, was one of the wealthiest in medieval Florence. Around 1285 Arnolfo di Cambio rebuilt the church which was then radically restructured in the seventeenth century when its facade was changed to face north in the direction of Via Alighieri. Traces of the old, thirteenth-century rear facade can still be seen in Via del Proconsolo.

The interior, following a Greek cross plan, has a carved Baroque ceiling replacing Arnolfo's painted wooden beams. Filippino Lippi's lovely *Apparition of the Virgin to St. Bernard* (around 1486) is to the left of the entrance; to the right, an altar front with a relief of the *Madonna and Child with Saints Leonardo and Lorenzo* by Mino da Fiesole (1464-1470) who was also the sculptor of the tomb of Bernardo Giugni (ca. 1466) around the corner and that of Ugo, Margrave of Tuscany, and son of the Badia's founder, in the arm of the cross to the left of the main altar.

Accessibility: Not accessible to wheelchairs. At the entrance in Via Alighieri there are two steps (20 centimeters [8 inches] each), then four more steps (17 centimeters [6 ¾ inches] each) with handrail into the Renaissance courtyard preceding the main door into the church.

Casa di Dante
Via Santa Margherita, 1
Tel: 055 219 416
Open: Temporarily closed for renovation
Admission: Charged

Description: Extensive restructuring promises to allow access to wheelchairs in this (1910) reconstruction of Dante's house. In the small Piazza di San Martino nearby is the much more interesting **Oratory of San Martino** once belonging to the parish church of the Alighieri, Dante's family (open 10:00-12:00; 15:00-17:00 every day except Sunday, holidays, and Friday afternoon. Two steps at entrance: 5 centimeters [2 inches] and 15 centimeters [6 inches]). In the fifteenth century, the small oratory was assigned to the *Compagnia dei Buonuomini,* a religious society who dedicated themselves to helping the *poveri vergognosi,* the poor who were too ashamed to beg. The charming late fifteenth-century frescoes painted inside by the circle of Ghirlandaio illustrate the good deeds of San Martino. One scene depicts the saint cutting his cloak in two to share with a beggar who was shivering from the cold. In

Italy Indian summer is known instead as *L'estate di San Martino* or Saint Martin's summer.

Accessibility: There are two steps at the entrance with double doors, both of which can be opened to allow a partial view of the small interior.

Palazzo Vecchio and the Museo dei Ragazzi
Piazza della Signoria
Tel: 055 276 8224
Open: Weekdays (except Thursday), 9:00-19:00; Thursday, 9:00-14:00; Sundays and holidays, 9:00-19:00
Admission: €6,00

Description: Originally built towards the end of the thirteenth century as a government palace according to a project by Arnolfo di Cambio, the *Palazzo della Signoria* was transformed into a sumptuous official residence when Duke Cosimo I moved his family there in 1540 as a symbolic act of renewed Medici power. In 1565, when he moved again, across the river to the Palazzo Pitti, to make way for his son and successor, Francesco I, the ducal palace became known as the "old palace" or *Palazzo Vecchio*. Today it is Florence's town hall, and although some of the most beautifully decorated apartments are occupied by the mayor, much of the palace has been turned into a museum.

Most of the decoration seen today in the palace dates to the architect and painter Giorgio Vasari's mid-sixteenth-century renovation project to convert the medieval government chambers into the Medici residence. Downstairs the walls of the courtyard inside the main entrance were decorated with scenes of Austrian cities in honor of Francesco's bride, Joan of Austria. For the audience hall upstairs, also known as the *Salone del '500*, Vasari designed an impressive wooden ceiling, ingeniously hung from the roof rafters, with painted panels depicting important events from Florentine history, and at the center, an apotheosis of the duke. Frescoed scenes of Florentine victories over Pisa and Siena are represented on the walls below, while a marble statue of *Victory* by Michelangelo exhalts the theme of conquest. Marble statues of Medici popes and dukes, including Cosimo and his sons, decorate the podium at the end of the room. Other rooms in the palace decorated by Vasari and his assistants include the exquisite tiny *Studiolo* or study of Francesco I and the apartments of Medici Pope Leo X on the main (second) floor (most rooms in the apartments are closed to the public); together with those of Cosimo's wife, Eleonora of Toledo, and the state rooms known as the *Quartieri degli Elementi* on the third floor. Additional rooms on this floor include the Priors' Chapel built in 1511, two government meeting chambers: the *Udienza* and *Sala dei Gigli* with Donatello's bronze statue of *Judith and the Holofernes,* as well as a map room decorated for Cosimo with a mid-sixteenth-century globe and maps of the known world.

Accessibility: The front entrance to the Palazzo Vecchio from Piazza della Signoria has six steps (no handrail). The wheelchair-accessible entrance is on the north side through the *Porta della Dogana* (behind the *Neptune* fountain). Both entrances are subject to a security check. There is a wheelchair-accessible ATM cash machine just inside the wheelchair-accessible entrance. The ticket office is located in the southeast corner of the courtyard (ramp at entrance). Entrance to the bookshop is by ramp to the right of ticket counter. To the left of the ticket counter are the reservation desk, accessible restroom, cloakroom, some rooms belonging to the Children's Museum, and the elevator to the main museum upstairs (elevator door width: 75 centimeters [29 ½ inches]; cabin width: 172 centimeters [67 ¾ inches]; cabin length: 109 centimeters [43 inches]). One manual wheelchair is available for use. The key to the accessible restroom and the wheelchair are kept in the cloakroom.

The main museum is located on the second and third floors and is reached either by monumental staircases (with handrails) or by the elevator located near the ticket office. On the second floor, there is a self-operable platform lift to the right of the podium in the **Salone del '500** for a closer look at the statues of the Medici.

Go through the glass doors at the entrance on the long side of the room for a partial glimpse of Vasari's Mannerist roller-coaster-like staircase. Entrance to Leo X's room (in the corner near the elevator bank) is reached by four steps (no handrails). The stair-climbing device you might see parked outside the elevator does not work. Steps lead up to the doorway into the **Studiolo** of Francesco I. Although the door is generally left open, you cannot enter the *Studiolo*, except with a special guided tour (not wheelchair accessible) arranged at the reservation desk downstairs.

Take the elevator to the third floor. Turn left outside the elevator for the **Quartiere degli Elementi**. Differences in levels between some of the rooms are negotiable by small ramps. There are two steps from the *Terrazza di Saturno* back into the *Sala degli Elementi*; retrace your path in order to leave this part of the palace. The balcony located to the right as you exit from the elevator leads to the grand duchess's apartments or **Quartiere di Eleonora** and narrows briefly to 74 centimeters (29 $1/8$ inches). Leaving Eleonora's apartments, the visit continues through the Priors' Chapel, the *Udienza*, the *Sala dei Gigli*, the *Cancelleria*, and the map room. Wheelchair users and people with limited mobility will then need to retrace this route to the elevator.

To reach the **Loeser Collection,** a bequest made to city in 1928 by the American art historian Charles Loeser which is located on the mezzanine level in the former apartments of Cosimo I's mother, Maria Salviati, go down the staircase located next to the *Sala dei Gigli*. The low steps (11 centimeters [4 ¼ inches] high) with handrail are divided into two flights of stairs by a landing. The staircase into the Loeser Collection has eight steps down with a handrail. The **battlements** are also reached from the third floor by the same staircase located next to the *Sala Dei Gigli* and involve three steep flights of stairs up (total of seventy-six steps:18 centimeters [7 ¼ inches] high).

Before leaving the palace, be sure to visit the courtyard on the ground floor at the Piazza della Signoria entrance. Irregular stone pavement is found in both courtyards. There are small lips at some doorway thresholds upstairs. Little seating is available except in the *Salone del '500*.

Comments: This is a huge palace and requires a minimum of two to three hours to see. Excellent guided tours are given (price of each tour is €2,00 in addition to the regular entrance ticket) to areas of the palace otherwise off limits to visitors, including the *Studiolo* of Francesco I and the attic for a view of the gigantic trusses that support the *Salone del '500* ceiling. Since these tours involve climbing many narrow, winding staircases without banisters, they are not accessible to wheelchairs or to people with limited mobility.

Museo dei Ragazzi (Children's Museum)
Tel: 055 276 8224 or 276 8558
Home Page: *www.museoragazzi.it*
Open: Every afternoon except Thursday when the Palazzo Vecchio is closed

Admission: By reservation only and in the company of an adult. Cost of ticket for children under seventeen is €2,00. Special prices are available for families.

Description: Visits are conducted in Italian and, by request, in English. The ground-floor activities include "La Stanza dei Giochi di Bia e Garzia" (The Playroom of Bia and Garzia, children of Cosimo I) which offers three different performances and one workshop. Most of these activities are suitable for small children between the ages of three and seven with one activity, "La Sfida fra il Mago della Luce a e il Mago dell'Ombra" (a performance involving the play between light and shadow) suitable for slightly older children between seven and eleven. Upstairs activities concerning costume and architecture are for children eight years and older.

Accessibility: Only the activities in the ground-floor rooms of the Children's Museum are accessible to wheelchair users. Other activities, located in upstairs rooms, involve steps. The history of costume activities, which include a performance in which the audience meets Duke Cosimo and his family, is held in one of the rooms of the Loeser Collection. On occasion, children in lightweight wheelchairs have been carried down the stairs to this part of the palace which is normally not accessible to wheelchairs. See above for description of accessibility.

Uffizi (accessible with assistance)
Piazzale degli Uffizi, 6
Tel: 055 238 8651
Home Page: *www.uffizi.firenze.it*
Open: Tuesday-Saturday, 8:15-18:50; Sundays and holidays, 8:30-18:50; closed on Monday
Admission: €8,50

Description: The Uffizi not only ranks together with the Louvre, the Hermitage, or London's National Gallery as one of the world's most famous art museums but is also the earliest museum in Europe to grant permission to visit its collections. Originally the building, begun around 1560 by Giorgio Vasari, was intended to house government offices. Around 1581 the top-floor, open loggia was closed in and transformed into a gallery, open to the public by special permission as early as 1591. The collection's earliest works included paintings by Raphael, Andrea del Sarto, Pontormo, and other Florentine artists, in addition to objects: weapons, maps, and scientific instruments. Laboratories for distilling perfumes and creating antidotes occupied the west wing together with a garden on the roof of the Loggia dei Lanzi where the museum café is now located. The Medici grand duke Ferdinando I enriched the collection with important pieces of antique sculpture that he had collected during his sojourn in Rome as cardinal at the papal court. In the seventeenth century, Vittoria della Rovere, bride of Ferdinando II, brought to the gallery, as part of her dowry, a large number of Venetian paintings as well as works by Raphael and the famous portraits of the duke and duchess of Urbino by Piero della

Francesca. Further Medici generations continued to make acquisitions, and in 1737 the last Medici, Anna Maria Luisa, stipulated that, upon her death, the entire collection would remain intact in the city of Florence and be opened as a public museum.

The vast collection, housed on the top floor (take elevator to level 3) together with the museum café, includes antique sculpture and paintings primarily from the twelfth through the eighteenth century. With the exception of the octagonal room known as the *Tribuna,* designed around 1584 to house the prized pieces of the Medici collection, the galleries are arranged chronologically and by school. Some of the most outstanding masterpieces in the east wing include a trio of *Enthroned Madonnas* by the medieval painters Duccio, Giotto, and Cimabue (room 2); Simone Martini's *Annunciation* painted for the cathedral in Siena (room 3); Gentile da Fabriano's *Adoration of the Magi* (room 6); the *Virgin and Child with Saint Anne* by Massacio, Piero della Francesca's Urbino portraits, and Paolo Uccello's *Battle of San Romano* (room 7); Botticelli's *Primavera* and *Birth of Venus* (room 10); Leonardo da Vinci's *Adoration of the Magi* and *Annunciation* and the *Baptism of Christ* by Verrocchio where Leonardo lent a hand in painting one of the angels (room 15); and some works by Durer and Mantegna (room 20).Continuing in the west wing are Michelangelo's *Holy Family* and Raphael's *Madonna of the Goldfinch* (room 25); works by Andrea del Sarto, Pontormo, and Rosso il Fiorentino (rooms 26 and 27); and Titian's *Venus of Urbino* (room 28). Some superb paintings by Rembrandt (room 37) and Rubens (room 41) point out that, although the majority of works are Italian with a logical emphasis on Florentine art, the collection also includes important paintings by leading European old masters. The drawing collection is located in the east wing on the *piano nobile* (take elevator to level 2). Entrance to the rooms used for temporary exhibitions located on level 2 is in the west wing. A shop selling books and gifts is located on the ground floor at the main entrance. Near future plans to construct a new entrance to the Uffizi (presently used as the main exit) will undoubtedly bring further changes and improvements to the museum's accessibility.

Accessibility: The **wheelchair-accessible entrance** to the museum portico is by a ramp located on the east side of the Uffizi at the corner of Via della Ninna opposite Palazzo Vecchio. Access to the ramp is difficult to negotiate and will require assistance. The level of the sidewalk at the entrance to the ramp in Via Della Ninna is 4 centimeters, just over 1 ½ inches above street level. Once on the sidewalk, you must make a 90-degree turn onto the ramp from the cramped space of the sidewalk which has a highly irregular stone pavement.

From the level of the portico, the wheelchair-accessible entrance is through the third door on the left. Note: The short ramp at this entrance has small lips both at the base (4 centimeters [approximately 1 ½ inches]) and top (5 centimeters [2 inches]). The stone pavement under the portico is extremely bumpy and uneven.

If you have made reservations to visit the museum through Firenze Musei, then proceed directly to the reservations desk which is located through the third to the last door on the left of the portico in the far (west) wing of the museum. Once you have picked up your tickets, you can take the larger elevator in the west wing to the galleries upstairs. (For description of this elevator see below.)

Four wheelchairs, available for loan, are stored in the cloakroom (*guardaroba*) located in the main hall inside the accessible entrance in the east wing.

Two self-operating small elevators, located to the left of the main staircase inside the ticket entrance in the east wing, are each capable of holding one wheelchair (door width: 64 centimeters [25 ¼ inches]; cabin width: 118 centimeters [46 ½ inches]; cabin depth: 139 centimeters [54 ¾ inches]). Push 2 for the Drawing Department exhibition space (*Gabinetto dei disegni*). Exiting from the elevator, first turn right, then left going through double wooden doors (each 48 centimeters [just under 19 inches wide]; both doors can be opened). Push 3 for the main galleries on the top floor.

A larger elevator is located in the west wing (elevator door width 90 centimeters [35 ½ inches]). This elevator is capable of holding at least two wheelchairs. A museum guard must accompany you if you wish to use this elevator.

The entire gallery of the Uffizi is accessible with the exception of the collection of artist's self-portraits in Vasari's corridor which is reached by a long and steep flight of stairs (admission by appointment only). In the *Tribuna* (room 18) visitors are confined to a corded-off walkway (sufficiently large enough for the passage of a wheelchair or scooter) which circles the room's perimeter. Scattered seating is found in the corridors of the east and west wings and in some galleries.

A **wheelchair-accessible restroom** is located on the top floor (level 3) in the west wing near the elevator between rooms 42 and 43. There is an adapted restroom in the temporary exhibition area (level 2) in the east wing, but to reach this restroom there are two steps (no ramp). To use these restrooms, you must ask a guard to unlock the door. The main restrooms on the top floor of the west wing of the gallery are not wheelchair accessible as they are located down one flight of stairs.

The museum café is located at the far end of the west wing. The platform lift to the right of the stairs at the entrance must be operated by museum personnel. Tables in the café are located outside on the terrace and in two other areas inside: in a separate lower room (down five steps) or on a balcony (up eleven steps). A table can be set up in the bar area upon request. A lowered credit card telephone is located near the café entrance at the top of the stairs next to the platform lift.

To leave the gallery or to visit the exhibitions on the lower floor, ask one of the guards stationed near the exit in the west wing to accompany you downstairs in the elevator. To return to street level, either backtrack to the ramp at the corner of Via della Ninna in the east wing or negotiate two steps at the end of the portico at the west-wing exit.

Temporary exhibitions are sometimes held on the ground floor of the Uffizi's west wing in the former *Regie poste*. The entrance has two steps approximately 13 centimeters (5 ½ inches) each.

Comments: To avoid waiting in line for hours, reservations are necessary to see this museum. If the top-floor, accessible restroom in the west wing is out of order, there is another one on the floor below in an area that is closed to the general public. To use this restroom, a museum guard must accompany you there with the elevator located in the west wing.

Mercato Nuovo
Piazza Mercato Nuovo (between Piazza della Repubblica and the Ponte Vecchio)
Open: Every day except Monday, 9:00-18:30

Description: The "new" market was designed between 1547 and 1551 by Giovanni Battista del Tasso just a stone's throw away from the "old" market which once occupied the site of present-day Piazza della Repubblica. At first silk and gold were sold under its arches. Later, in the nineteenth century, this was known as the "straw market" when straw hats, famous throughout Europe, were sold there. The market is also called the ."market of the *porcellino*," named after the bronze statue of a boar, a sixteenth-century copy of a Greek original now housed in the Uffizi Gallery, which is located on its southern side.

Accessibility: The market loggia is accessible by several different ramps located on the west side of the piazza.

Towards the Arno

Museo di Storia della Scienza (accessible with assistance)
Piazza dei Giudici, 1
Tel: 055 293 493 (recording in Italian and English); 055 265 311
E-mail: *imss@imss.fi.it*
Home Page: *www.imss.fi.it*
Open: Summer (June 1-Sept 30)—Monday, Wednesday, Thursday, Friday, 9:30-17:00; Tuesday and Saturday, 9:30-13:00; closed on Sunday; open last Thursday of June and August and first Thursday of July and September, evenings 21:00-23:00.
Winter (Oct 1-May 31)—Monday, Wednesday, Thursday, Friday,

Saturday, 9:30-17:00; Tuesday, 9:30-13:00; second Sunday of the month, 10:00-13:00; otherwise closed on Sunday
Admission: €6,50

Description: This world-famous collection of scientific instruments offers a refreshing alternative to painting and sculpture. The 1° *piano* (second floor) rooms hold objects from the fifteenth to seventeenth centuries once belonging to the Medici: compasses, astrolabes, sundials, globes, and telescopes, including two made by Galileo. The 2° *piano* (third floor) rooms contain objects from the Lorraine dynasty (eighteenth to nineteenth centuries) ranging from mechanical clocks to a fascinating, if somewhat explicit, display of anatomical wax models related to childbirth, used in the teaching of medicine in Florence at the end of the eighteenth century. Written descriptions in English of the objects on exhibition are available to borrow in many of the rooms.

Accessibility: There is a high sidewalk in front of entrance with curb cut at crosswalk near the river. Entrance has three steps. Ring doorbell (height: 134 centimeters [52 ¾ inches]) for portable ramps (width: 74 centimeters [29 inches]). Ticket office is on left inside the entrance. Be sure to take a free museum guide.

Itinerary: The museum is laid out on two floors: the 1° and 2° *piano* (second and third floors) are each reached by a different elevator (elevator door widths: 80 centimeters [31 ½ inches]; cabin widths: 110 centimeters [43 ¼ inches]; cabin lengths: 140 centimeters [55 ⅛ inches]). Take Elevator A in entrance lobby to the 2° *piano* (third floor) galleries. An accessible restroom is located on this floor (WC 51 centimeters [20 inches] high with retractable grab bars to right and left). Elevator B to the 1° *piano* (second floor) galleries is located on the lower level (four steps down) reached by stair lift (width: 70 centimeters [27 ½ inches]; length: 85 centimeters [33 ½ inches]; capacity: 190 kilograms [418 pounds]). To reach the 2 ° *piano* from the 1° *piano*, take Elevator B up again and exit from elevator for a second stair lift (dimensions as given above) to the 2° *piano*. Once you reach the 2° *piano*, you can return directly to the ground floor with Elevator A. Three flights of stairs with handrails connect each floor.

Around Via Tornabuoni

Museo Ferragamo (not accessible)
Via Tornabuoni, 2
Tel: 055 336 0456
Open: Monday-Friday, 9:00-13:00 and 14:00-18:00
No Admission Fees

Description: Ferragamo was a cobbler from a town outside Naples who went to Hollywood and made it big, designing sandals for Cecil B. DeMille's *Cleopatra* and decking out stars like Greta Garbo in beautifully designed, custom-made footwear. In 1927, when he came back to Italy, he chose to work in Florence, a city where artisans were known for their outstanding craftsmanship. Of the over ten thousand examples in the museum archives, a select group of shoes, designed for clients such as the Duchess of Windsor, Marilyn Monroe, Bridget Bardot, and Madonna, are displayed in the museum's four rooms.

Accessibility: Not accessible to wheelchairs. There are two steps at the main entrance at street level. The museum is located on the *primo piano* (second floor) and is reached by four flights of stairs (for a total of eighty steps) or by a tiny elevator (door width 55 centimeters [21 ⁵/₈ inches]) with two steps from the elevator to the museum entrance on the second floor.

Palazzo Davanzati (entrance accessible for manual wheelchairs only with assistance)
Via Porta Rossa, 13
Tel: 055 238 8610
Open: The palace is presently closed for renovation, and only the entrance loggia is visible.
Admission: Free to see the loggia

Description: Built by a wealthy merchant family in the mid-fourteenth century, Palazzo Davanzati has been open to the public as a museum since the early 1900s. The upstairs rooms, some decorated with painted, fictive tapestries, are furnished with antiques from the fifteenth and sixteenth centuries to represent a typical Renaissance interior.

Accessibility: There is a step at the entrance door into the loggia: 13 centimeters (5 $^1/_8$ inches) up; 5.5 centimeters (2 ¼ inches) down to floor level. Hopefully, this most recent renovation will improve accessibility to the upper three floors.

Palazzo Strozzi (assistance advised)
Piazza Strozzi
Tel: 055 288 342. For information on the exhibitions, call 055 264 5155
Open: The courtyard is always visible when the library, located inside the palace, is open: Monday and Friday, 9:00-13:00, and Tuesday, Wednesday, Thursday, 9:00-18:00; and otherwise, for more extensive time, when there is an exhibition. Opening times for exhibitions vary.
Admission: Free to view the courtyard. Admission is charged for the exhibitions periodically held upstairs on the main floor.

Description: The wealthy Strozzi family had been bankers to the kings of Naples and their palace, begun in 1489 and completed some fifty years later, was, at the time of its construction, the largest in Renaissance Florence. Its design, inspired by the Palazzo Medici, represented the quintessence of Florentine palace architecture: a symmetrical square built around a central courtyard with a rusticated stone facade pierced by rounded, arched windows and a central door and crowned by a classically inspired cornice.

Accessibility: Two ill-fitting short wooden ramps lead from the sidewalk level into the palace courtyard at the main entrance facing Piazza Strozzi. The ticket office and the elevators to the upper floors are located on the left side of the courtyard. Take the larger elevator (on the left) to the main floor (1° *piano*). The elevator door pulls out. Open door width is 79 centimeters (31 inches); cabin width is 139 centimeters (54 ¾ inches); cabin depth is 114 centimeters, just under 45 inches. There is a ramp into the women's restroom located upstairs on the main floor (WC has retractable grab bars, on the right and left, with room for right transfer). The men's restroom (one step) also has an adapted WC, but at the time of inspection there was no ramp at the entrance to this restroom. There is a small ramp into the bookstore. Scattered seating can usually be found in the exhibition rooms. A third accessible restroom is located off the courtyard on the ground floor; ask at the ticket office for the key (low WC 42 centimeters [16 ½ inches]; grab bars; right transfer).

Santissimi Apostoli (not accessible)
Borgo SS Apostoli at Piazza del Limbo
Tel: 055 290 642
Open: 10:00-12:00; 15:30-17:00; Sunday, 10:00-13:00
No Admission Fees

Description: The Church of the "Holy Apostles" is a Romanesque structure contemporary with the Baptistery and dating to the latter half of the eleventh century. The Renaissance entrance portal is by Benedetto da Rovezzano. Despite later alterations, including the rebuilt side chapels and a 1930s restoration, the dark, suggestive interior with its painted timber ceiling still remains one of the earliest and finest church interiors in Florence. Two capitals in the nave nearest the entrance are spoils from the first-century-AD Roman baths in nearby Via delle Terme.

Accessibility: Not accessible to wheelchairs. The small piazza in front of the church, once a graveyard for unbaptized infants, is reached either from Borgo SS Apostoli (five steps down from the street level to the piazza) or from an alleyway leading from Lungarno Acciaioli (two steps down to the piazza). There are two steps up, then two down at the church entrance.

Santa Trinita
Piazza Santa Trinita
Tel: 055 216 912
Open: 8:00-12:00; 16:00-18:00; Sunday, 16:00-18:00
No Admission Fees

Description: Santa Trinita is the mother church of the Vallombrosan
Order founded in the eleventh century by a Florentine nobleman,
Giovanni Gualberto. A typical Italian *pastiche* with Gothic interior
and Late Renaissance facade by Bernardo Buontalenti, the main
attraction of the church are the frescoes painted by Ghirlandaio
(1483-1486), located in the second chapel to the right of the
main altar, showing the life of St. Francis against a background of
Renaissance Florence. "St. Francis Receiving the Order of the Rule"
appears complete with members of the Medici family and Francesco
Sassetti, patron of the chapel, and his sons in front of the Loggia
dei Lanzi in Piazza della Signoria. Piazza Santa Trinita forms the
background to the scene of the "Miracle of the Child," seen falling
from a palace window on the left and brought back to life by St.
Francis.

Accessibility: Wheelchair-accessible entrance is through the right
door of the main facade. Nave is barrier free with skid-free short
ramps to the presbytery area. There are six steps up to Ghirlandaio's
Sassetti Chapel, but the frescoes can be seen from the nave level. A
coin-operated light box to illuminate the chapel is located at the
top of the steps inside the chapel on the left wall.

Santa Maria Novella

This neighborhood, extending west of Via Tornabuoni to Porta a Prato and from the Santa Maria Novella railroad station to the Arno, is dominated by the Dominican Convent and **Church of Santa Maria Novella**. Piazza Santa Maria Novella, flanked on one side by the church and on the other by the fifteenth-century convalescent hospital of San Paolo, was once the scene of Renaissance horse races. Today it is a popular gathering place for the city's growing immigrant population. To the east in Piazza San Pancrazio is the **Museo di Marino Marini** with nearby **Palazzo Rucellai,** home of Giovanni Rucellai who commissioned the Renaissance facade of the Church of Santa Maria Novella. Closer to the river in Borgo Ognissanti is the **Church of Ognissanti** with **Ghirlandaio's** famous *Last Supper* in the adjacent convent refectory. In this neighborhood you'll find a little bit of everything: from the tourist hotels clustered around the streets leading to the station, to the elegant antique shops in Via de' Fossi and Borgo Ognissanti, and chic boutiques in Via Vigna Nuova.

Mobility

Getting There

Wheelchair-accessible electric **Bus D** follows a circular route leaving the RR station (bus stop is opposite the taxi stand on the "Arrivals" side of the station) and heading across the river to Piazza Ferrucci. Stops include Via Curtatone (for the American Consulate), Borgo San Frediano, Ponte Vecchio, and Piazza Ferrucci. Return trip from Piazza Ferrucci makes stops at Palazzo Pitti, Piazza Santo Spirito, and Piazza del Carmine before returning to the RR station.

Electric Bus A (direction "Beccaria") leaving from the station (bus stop is outside the "Departures" entrance) makes stops at the bottom of Piazza Santa Maria Novella, in Borgo Ognissanti, in Via del Parione next to the Church of Santa Trinita, turning left down Via Tornabuoni. On the return trip from Piazza Beccaria stops include Via Vigna Nuova (near Palazzo Rucellai), Via delle Belle Donne (for Piazza Santa Maria Novella), the station.

Electric Bus B (direction "Piave") runs along the edge of the Santa Maria Novella neighborhood near the river and makes a circular route connecting Ponte della Vittoria near the Cascine Park, to Piazza Piave. Stops include the American Consulate, the Santa Trinita Church, Ponte Vecchio, the Uffizi.

Getting Around

With the exception of Piazza Santa Maria Novella, there are no extensive pedestrian zones in this area, and major streets have normal traffic flow. The most wheelchair-friendly routes are located in Via degli Avelli, from Via de'Panzani along the side of the Church of Santa Maria Novella into the piazza; the west side of Via de'Fossi, leading from the Piazza Santa Maria Novella to Piazza Goldoni; the south side of Borgo Ognissanti, from Piazza Goldoni to Piazza Ognissanti; and Via della Vigna Nuova.

If you are heading for the center of town from the RR station, in order to avoid the busy traffic circle outside the station, you may want to take the underground pedestrian gallery. The elevator to the gallery and to the parking lot is located in the station's main ticket hall opposite the ticket counters. From the elevator, turn left into the gallery, following it around the corner and then straight to the end where you will find a ramp on the left leading to Piazza dell'Unità. This ramp is fairly steep and can be slippery when wet. Once you exit from the gallery, take Via Panzani for Piazza del Duomo which is about ten minutes away.

Taxi stands are located at the RR station to the right as you exit from the "Arrivals" side of the station, at the bottom of Piazza

Santa Maria Novella near Via della Scala and in Piazza dell'Unità on the way to the Duomo.

Ample **designated parking** for those with disability parking permits is located in the parking garage under the RR station. Enter from Piazza della Stazione, proceed straight through the ticket gate to a second gate for this reserved area. There are elevators up to the level of the station and the underground commercial gallery. You are eligible for free parking if you show your permit to the cashier upon leaving. For further details, see pp. 205-206 in "Transportation." To reach the underground garage from the *viali* take either Via S. Caterina d'Alessandria, then Via Nazionale or Via Diacceto, then Via Alamanni.

Except for the above-mentioned streets which lead to the station and the underground parking lot, **you will need permission to drive in most streets in this neighborhood which is part of the ZTL** (Limited Traffic Zone). For further information, see "Driving Around" in the chapter on "Transportation."

What the Neighborhood Has to Offer

The **American Consulate** is located at Lungarno Vespucci, 38 (Tel. No. 055 266 951). Nearby in Corso Italia is the **Teatro Comunale**, the city's main concert hall. The **British Consulate** is found at Lungarno Corsini, 2 (Tel. No. 055 284 133) near the Santa Trinita Bridge. American and British books are sold at the **BM Bookshop** (Borgo Ognissanti, 4/r; Tel. No. 055 294 575). Despite the heavy hotel concentration, this neighborhood does not offer much choice in wheelchair-accessible accommodations or places to eat. **Osteria N.1** (Via del Moro, 18/20; closed on Sunday; 8-centimeter [3 ¼-inch] step at entrance; accessible restroom) offers Tuscan/Venetian cuisine. **Coco Lezzone** (Via Parioncino, 26/r; Tel. No. 055 287178; closed on Sunday and Tuesday evening; one step at entrance 10 centimeters [4 inches] from narrow sidewalk; no accessible restroom); **Il Latini** (Via dei Palchetti, 6/r; Tel. No. 055 210 916; closed on Monday; accessible restroom), and **Marione** (Via della Spada, 27/r; Tel. No. 055

214 756; closed on Sunday) are excellent places to eat and serve hearty, traditional Florentine food. **La Rotonda**, popular with the younger crowd, is a lively place in the evenings to drink beer and eat pizza. A **tourist information office** is located in Piazza della Stazione, 4. The office is located down a short flight of stairs, and although there is a platform lift (with no call bell), most of the staff does not seem to have been trained to operate it.

Accessibility Checklist

The following list contains places which are accessible to people in wheelchairs.

Accommodations

- Hotel Kraft

Places to Eat

- Coco Lezzone
  Entrance has one step (10 centimeters [4 inches]) with a 10-centimeter (4-inch) curb on the sidewalk in front of the door. (Power wheelchairs have been known to enter this restaurant.)
- Il Latini
- La Rotonda
- Marione
  Five centimeters (2 inches) at threshold; no accessible restroom.
- McDonald's
  There are two of them: one is inside the station (tables are located upstairs and are not accessible to wheelchairs); the other (with accessible restroom) is directly across the street from the "Arrivals" entrance to the station. Accessible entrance is at Via Valfonda 25/r.
- Osteria N.1
- Self-Service Restaurant at the RR station

Accessible Restrooms

- Il Latini
- McDonald's in Via Valfonda, 25/r
- Osteria N. 1
- Museo Marino Marini
- Santa Maria Novella RR station (next to track 5)
  WC has retractable grab bar to left, vertical grab bar, and room for transfer to right.
- Commercial gallery under the Santa Maria Novella RR station
  Heading towards Piazza dell'Unità there is a public restroom located on the right beyond the Internet point. Entrance is not level, and the accessible small restroom is suitable for manual wheelchairs only. Small fee.

Banks

- Monte dei Paschi di Siena, Agenzia 19
  Tel: 055 260 8812
  Located in the underground gallery of the RR station opposite the fountain.
  Ring to enter through accessible door.

- Istituto Bancario San Paolo di Torino
  Tel: 055 282 619
  Located inside the RR station in the main hall opposite the tracks.
  Ring doorbell at the emergency exit to the left of the ATM machine.

Consulates

- American Consulate
  Lungarno Vespucci, 38
  Tel: 055 266 951

The consulate is not accessible to wheelchairs. Call ahead of time to make an appointment, and the consul or consulate personnel will meet you at the entrance.

- British Consulate
  Lungarno Corsini, 2
  Tel: 055 284 133
  Located upstairs. There is one step to the elevator. Elevator dimensions are door width: 54 centimeters (21 ½ inches); cabin width: 120 centimeters (47 ¼ inches); cabin depth: 80 centimeters (31 ½ inches).

Internet Points

- Internet Train
  Located in the underground gallery of the RR station.
  Tel: 055 239 9720
  Open: Monday-Friday, 9:00-20:00; Saturday and Sunday, 11:00-20:00
  Take the stair lift on the stairs at the "Arrivals" entrance opposite Via Valfonda. Internet Train is located on your left just a few meters down the gallery as you head in the direction of the Duomo. If the stair lift is not working, take the elevator located inside the station ticket hall opposite the ticket counters. Turn left out of the elevator, then right at the fountain opposite the stairs.

Pharmacies

- Farmacia Comunale n. 13
  Stazione di Santa Maria Novella
  Tel: 055 216 761
  Located inside the "Arrivals" entrance on the left. Open twenty-four hours.
- Farmacia della Stazione
  Via Panzani, 65/r
  Tel: 055 265 4326
- Farmacia Sodoni

Via dei Banchi, 18/r
Tel: 055 211 159
Two-centimeter (¾-inch) lip at threshold. Also sells homeo-
pathic remedies.

Santa Maria Novella

Monuments

1. American Consulate
2. British Consulate
3. Church of Ognissanti and Cenacolo
4. Church of Santa Maria Novella and Museum
5. Marino Marini Museum
6. Cappella Rucellai
7. Palazzo Rucellai

Places to Eat

1. Coco Lezzone
2. Marione
3. Il Latini
4. Osteria N. 1
5. La Rotonda
6. McDonald's

Accommodations

1. Hotel Kraft

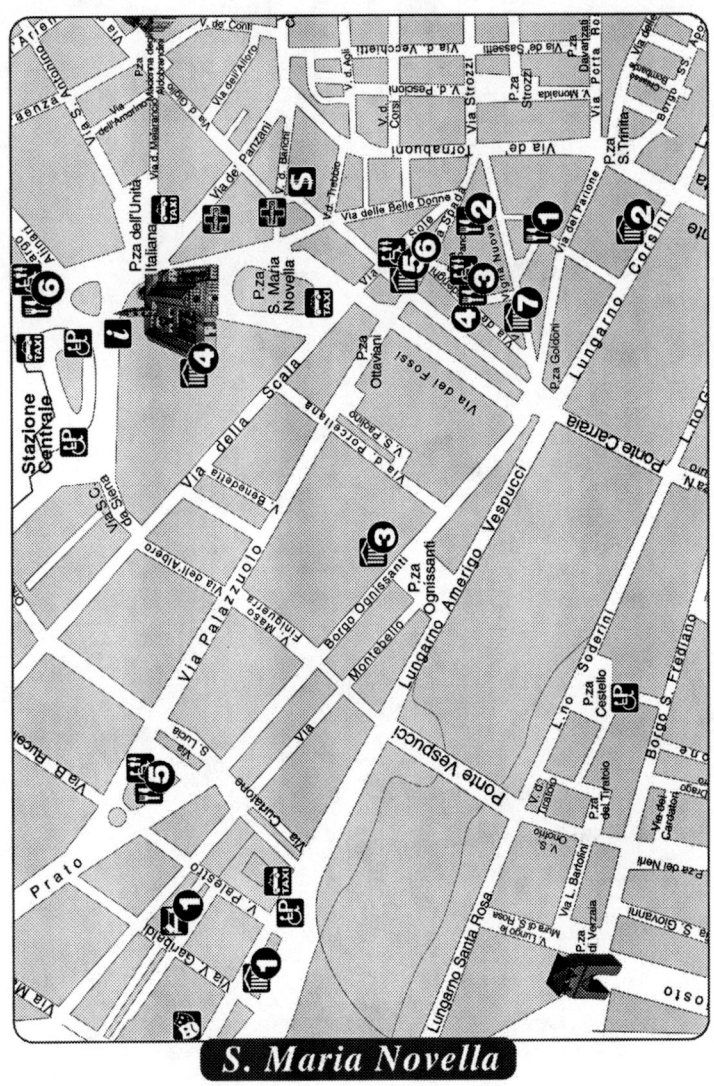

S. Maria Novella

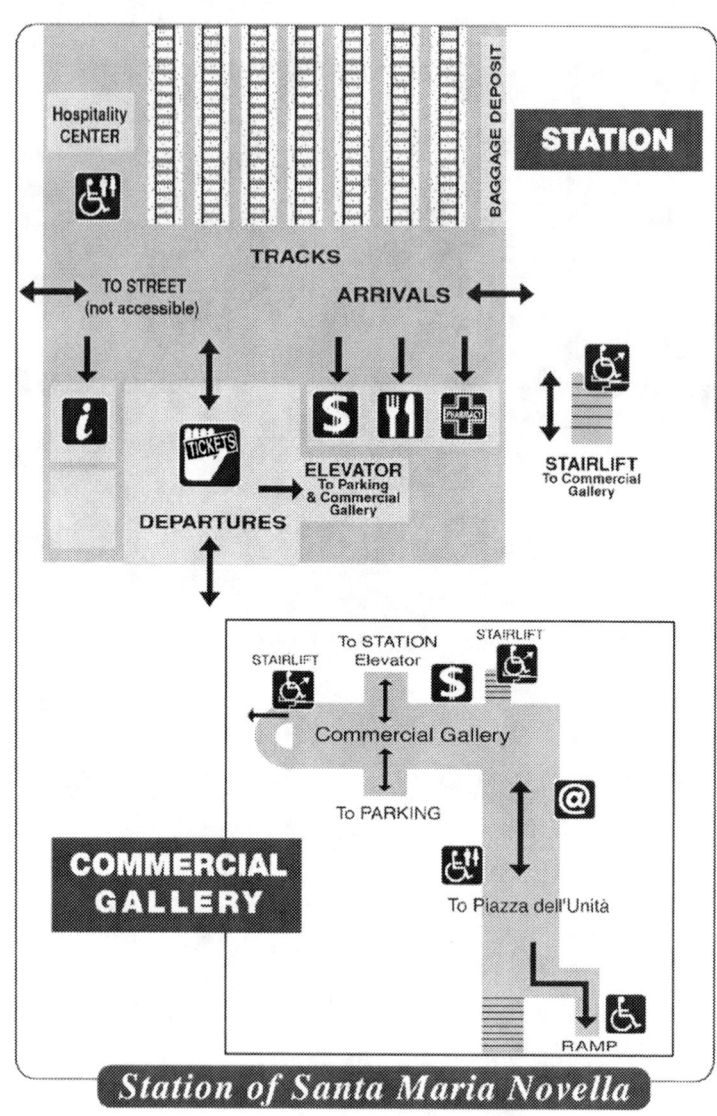

Station of Santa Maria Novella

What to See

Church of Santa Maria Novella
Piazza Santa Maria Novella
Tel: 055 282 187
Open: Monday-Thursday and Saturday, 9:30-17:00; Friday and Sunday, 13:00-17:00
Admission: €2,50

Description: The two great religious orders in thirteenth-century Florence, the Franciscans and the Dominicans, were each responsible for building an important church. The Franciscans, devoted to the poor, built their church in the working-class neighborhood of Santa Croce. The Dominicans, whose name literally means "hounds of the lord" *(domini canes),* set out to combat heresy; Santa Maria Novella is their church. The present church was begun in 1246, but by the fifteenth century, its facade was still incomplete. Around 1458 Leon Battista Alberti, architect of the nearby Rucellai Palace, was commissioned by the wealthy wool merchant Giovanni Rucellai to complete the facade. Alberti incorporated the string of medieval wall tombs and side portals on the lower story and, inspired by the design of the Romanesque Church of San Miniato which overlooks Florence, created a masterpiece of Renaissance harmonic proportions. The severe Gothic interior and didactic nature of the many of the decorations inside the church attest to the order's militant and dogmatic role in spreading church doctrine. Massacio's recently restored *Trinità* (ca. 1425) in the left nave recalls St. Augustine's treatise on God as one nature in three persons, a theme dear to the Dominican order whose calendar year began on the feast day of the Trinity. Two donors kneel outside the first architectural perspective to appear in a Renaissance painting according to Brunelleschi's principles. The aged Virgin, opposite St. John, points didactically to the crucified Christ with God the Father above and the Holy Spirit, looking more like a white handkerchief than a dove, above Christ's head. A

Crucifix by Giotto hangs in the center of the nave; a wooden crucifix by Brunelleschi is in the chapel to the left of the main altar. The cycle of stories from the lives of the Virgin and St. John the Baptist by Ghirlandaio (1485) and his workshop, which included the young Michelangelo, are in the choir. Filippino Lippi worked in the Strozzi Chapel next door on scenes from the life of St. Philip and St. John the Evangelist (1487-1502) where the frenzied agitation of the figures, carried over into the decorative detail, anticipates the tensions and ambiguities of the later Mannerist style. The Rucellai Chapel further to the right once housed Duccio's *Maestà,* today in the Uffizi.

Accessibility: Entrance to the church is from a raised podium reached by a short flight of steps and made accessible by two ramps: one to the right, the other to the left of the podium. The left ramp has a small lip at the base: 2 centimeters (¾ inch). Go into the cloister on the right side of the church, then straight ahead to the ramped entrance. Inside the church, the main nave is free of barriers with a ramp leading to the raised presbytery area. The transept chapels, the choir decorated by Ghirlandaio behind the main altar, and the sacristy with bookstore all have steps and are not accessible to wheelchair users. Nevertheless, all the side chapels have good visibility from the presbytery except for the chapels at the ends of the transepts and one of the most beautiful of Ghirlandaio's scenes, the *Birth of St. John the Baptist,* with the extraordinary, windswept figure of a handmaiden bearing a plate of fruit on her head, is still visible from the left side of the main altar.

Museo of Santa Maria Novella
Piazza Santa Maria Novella (Wheelchair-accessible entrance is through the door of the Fratellanza Militare, Piazza Santa Maria Novella, 18.)
Tel: 055 282 187
Open: Saturday-Thursday, 9:00-16:30; Sunday, 9:00-14:00; closed on Friday
Admission: €2,60

Description: The museum is on the ground floor of the Convent of Santa Maria Novella, located to the left of the church. Paolo Uccello's frescoes, faded shadows of a once-vivid green monochrome, decorate the walls of the *Chiostro Verde* or "green courtyard." The artificial spatial constructions of the Old Testament *Deluge* and *Drunkenness of Noah* reflect the artist's passion for exploring Renaissance perspective. Dominican doctrine sets the theme for Andrea di Firenze's fourteenth-century decoration of the chapter house, more popularly known as the Spanish Chapel after it was designated in the sixteenth century as place of worship for members of the Spanish community headed by the wife of Grand Duke Cosimo de' Medici, Eleonora of Toledo. The refectory completes the museum with a collection of liturgical vestments and objects and, in the antechamber, fragments of heads of Old Testament prophets from the circle of Andrea Orcagna, which once decorated the ribs of the ceiling vaults behind the church's main altar.

Accessibility: There are six steps at the main entrance. The wheelchair-accessible entrance is through Piazza S. Maria Novella, 18. Ring bell and proceed to front door of museum. The guard will place a portable ramp at the entrance which has one step down (16 centimeters [6 ¼ inches]). **No accessible restroom.**

Museo Marino Marini
Piazza San Pancrazio
Tel: 055 219 432
Open: Monday, Wednesday-Saturday, 10:00-17:00; Sunday and Tuesday closed; closed on Saturday in June, July, September, and for the month of August.
Admission: €4,00

Description: Leon Battista Alberti designed the former Church of San Pancrazio now converted into the Museo Marino Marini. The collection is dedicated entirely to the work of one of Italy's most important modern artists, Marino Marini (1901-1980), best known for his sculptures developed on the horse-and-rider theme. Temporary exhibits of twentieth-century artists are held in the former crypt.

Accessibility: The entrance has six steps, no handrail, and a **stair lift** for wheelchairs to the right of the porch (width: 70 centimeters [27 ½ inches]; length: 73 centimeters [28 ¾ inches]; capacity: 130 kilograms [286 pounds]). There is an **accessible restroom** (WC 40 centimeters [15 ¾ inches] high; grab bars to left and rear; space for right transfer; the sink has an unwrapped metal pipe). An **elevator** goes to all floors (door width: 120 centimeters [47 ¼ inches]; cabin depth: 100 centimeter [39 ³/₈ inches]; cabin width: 183 centimeters [72 inches]). Guided tours, scheduled in advance, are available in English for visitors with visual impairments (for information see chapter on "Museums, Music, Movies, and Sports"). Seating is found throughout the museum.

Comments: This museum has generally good accessibility, but wheelchair users should stay away from the hazardous narrow balconies opposite the elevator banks on the first and second floors. Some prints and drawings are in high glass cases and not visible from the level of a wheelchair.

Palazzo Rucellai
Via Vigna Nuova, 18
The palace cannot be visited.

Description: Palazzo Rucellai was the home of the wealthy merchant, Giovanni Rucellai, whose family grew rich from importing a special purplish red dye from Majorca. His palace was designed in 1444 by Alberti, architect of the facade of nearby Santa Maria Novella. Alberti's design was somewhat an anomaly in local palace architecture with its use of the classical orders neatly dividing up the facade. Their progression from the simple to the elaborate: ground floor, Doric; *piano nobile,* Ionic; and top floor, Corinthian, followed the same progression of orders used for the Colosseum and demonstrate how attentive the Renaissance architect was to ancient Roman architecture. Across the street, the **Rucellai Loggia** was both an outdoor waiting room for Rucellai's business associates and a place to gather for conversation. The **Cappella Ruccellai** (in Via della Spada), built 1461-1467, is also by Alberti and contains a replica of the Holy Sepulchre in Jerusalem. The chapel is open only sporadically and has three high steps at the entrance. Tactile tours are offered by appointment by VIVAT. (For information see chapter on "Museums, Music, Movies, and Sports.")

Ognissanti (accessible with assistance)
Piazza Ognissanti
Open: 8:00-12:30; 17:00-19:30
Admission: Free

Description: The original Church of the Ognissanti was built in the thirteenth century by the *Umiliati,* monks from Lombardy who were first responsible for developing the wool industry in Florence. The facade is a faithful nineteenth-century copy of a seventeenth-century facade by Nigetti. In the interior in the right nave you'll find a *St. Augustine in His Study* by Botticelli who is also buried in the church. Directly across the nave is a *St. Jerome* by Ghirlandaio (both ca. 1480). In an early fresco by Ghirlandaio of the *Madonna of Mercy* protecting members of the Vespucci family (right nave), Amerigo, for whom America was named, is supposedly the young boy who appears between the Madonna and the man in the dark cape.

Accessibility: There is one step at the entrance to the church foyer (up 9 centimeters [3 ½ inches], then 3.5 centimeters [1 ¼ inches] down to floor level). The door into the church measures 71 centimeters (28 inches). The nave of the church is all on one level with the exception of the raised presbytery.

Cenacolo di Ognissanti (not accessible but can be viewed from a distance)
Borgo Ognissanti, 42
Information: 348 6450390
Open: 9:00-12:00, Monday, Tuesday, Saturday
Admission: Free

Description: Christ and the twelve apostles sit at a long table against a bright background of predatory birds soaring over lemon and cypress trees in Ghirlandaio's *Last Supper* (1480). Laden with symbolic imagery down to the griffins embroidered on the tablecloth, which stand for the dual—divine and human—nature of Christ, the fresco is similar to the one the artist painted at the Convent of San Marco.

Accessibility: The door to the *Cenacolo* is located to the left of the church facade. There is a short ramp at the entrance to the courtyard from the entrance foyer. Go around the courtyard to the far end where you see the double doors (61 centimeters [24 inches] each; both doors can be opened) at the entrance to the refectory vestibule which has a 3-centimeter (just over one inch) rise at the threshold. Once inside the vestibule, there are two steps into the refectory (each about 13 centimeters [5 ¼ inches]). Seating is available in front of the fresco. There is **no accessible restroom**.

Comments: The fresco is visible, although at a distance, from the refectory door.

San Lorenzo

The San Lorenzo neighborhood traditionally is Medici territory. Their impressive family home, **Palazzo Medici Riccardi**, dominates Via Cavour, the main street running north from Piazza del Duomo to Piazza San Marco. In the piazza behind the palace stands **San Lorenzo**, their parish church, a rich complex including the **Laurentian Library,** and the **Old and New Sacristies** and **Cappella dei Principi**, the private chapels where important Medici family members were buried.

Today the streets and piazza surrounding the church are filled with shops and open market stalls selling shoes, leather goods, inexpensive clothing, and tourist souvenirs. A covered market in nearby **Piazza del Mercato Centrale** sells everything from meat and fish, to wine, cheese, and fresh pasta on the ground floor and fruit, vegetables, and flowers upstairs. Further west Via Nazionale connects Piazza Indipendenza to the station.

Mobility

Getting There

Wheelchair-accessible Buses 7 and 23 coming from the station make stops in Via Martelli close to the Medici Palace. From the direction of Piazza San Marco, both buses stop in Via Martelli near Piazza del Duomo.

Getting Around

Much of the San Lorenzo area is pedestrian. This includes Borgo San Lorenzo (the main street leading from Piazza San Giovanni to

Piazza San Lorenzo), Piazza San Lorenzo, Via dell'Ariento up to Via Nazionale, and the streets to the side of the covered market. Borgo San Lorenzo and the first section of the street market along the front, side, and rear of the church are less wheelchair friendly than the stretches in Via dell'Ariento towards Via Nazionale which have new pavement. Most of the small side streets in the market area have bumpy stone pavement and narrow sidewalks without curb cuts.

Nearest **taxi stands** are in Via de'Pecori near Piazza San Giovanni and in Piazza dell'Unità near the station.

Four designated parking spaces are located in the twenty-four-hour parking garage underneath the covered *Mercato Centrale di San Lorenzo*. To reach the garage from the *viali*, take Via S. Caterina d'Alessandria to Via Nazionale, turn left in Via Guelfa, then immediately right in Via Panicale, left in Via Taddea, and right in Via Rosina into the piazza where straight ahead you will see the entrance to the parking garage. There is an elevator up to the market from the garage. After the market closes at 14:00 (2 p.m.), wheelchairs must enter and exit the garage using the car ramps. There is no charge if you show your disability permit to the attendant. To reach the garage, follow the above-described route otherwise **driving in this part of this town, which is part of the ZTL (Limited Traffic Zone), requires special permission.** See "Driving Around" in the chapter on "Transportation" for further details.

What the Neighborhood Has to Offer

A number of casual restaurants in Piazza del Mercato Centrale have outdoor seating in warm weather. Almost all outside seating is on a raised platform and involves one step. If you should choose one of these, but need a wheelchair-accessible restroom, there is a decent and clean **public wheelchair-accessible restroom** just around the corner in Via della Stufa, 25 (small fee). **Da Garibaldi** is the one restaurant in the piazza with an accessible restroom, with outdoor seating (one step) and level entrance. **Nerbone**, inside the covered market on the ground floor near the wheelchair-accessible entrance in Via dell'Ariento, serves lunch and is a good place to rub shoulders with the local market workers. **Nannini**, a busy coffee bar serving typical pastries from Siena (with wheelchair-accessible restroom), is located in Via Borgo San Lorenzo, the street leading into the market area from the Duomo; on the same side of the street is the self-service restaurant **Spleen Café** (accessible restroom). Further afield in Via Guelfa 81/r, west of Via Nazionale, **Trattoria La Gratella** (accessible restroom) offers a glutten-free menu.

Most of the shops in the area around the market sell inexpensive shoes and clothing, including secondhand togs and American army surplus items. A **tourist information office** is located in Via Cavour 1/r near the Medici Palace.

Accessibility Checklist

The following list contains information on various places which are accessible to wheelchairs.

Accommodations

- Hotel Botticelli
- Hotel Galileo
- Hotel il Guelfo Bianco
- Ostello Archi Rossi

Places to Eat

Several places to eat in Borgo San Lorenzo also have accessible restrooms, including the Ristorante Nuti (not the pizzeria on the opposite side of the street) and Giannino in San Lorenzo. However, their entrances are extremely difficult to negotiate due to placement of outside tables and narrow sidewalks.

- Da Garibaldi
  Narrow sidewalk in front of main entrance.

- Spleen Café
- La Gratella
- Nerbone
  Lunch only. Located inside the covered market.
- Nannini
- McDonald's in Via Cavour

Accessible restrooms

- Palazzo Medici
- Mercato Centrale di San Lorenzo
  Open: 7:00-14:00
- Via della Stufa, 25
  Open: 10:00-18:00; 9:00-19:00 in summer. One step at entrance. Ring bell for attendant to place ramp. The bathroom is spacious, but the distance of the fixed grab bars to the right of the WC will cause difficulty for some users. Ample space for left transfer. Cost €0,60.
- Da Garibaldi
  Grab bars. Space for left transfer.
- Spleen Café
  Grab bars. Space for right transfer.
- La Gratella
- Nannini
  WC has fixed grab bar on left wall; retractable bar on right with space for transfer.

Banks

- Cassa di Risparmio, Branch 6
  Via Nazionale, 93/95/r
  Tel: 055 261 041
  Ring bell. Wheelchair-accessible entrance is an emergency exit.

Pharmacies

- Farmacia del Mercato Centrale (opposite the covered market)
  Via dell'Ariento, 87/r
  Tel: 055 214 070

San Lorenzo

Monuments

1. Church of San Lorenzo
2. Cappelle Medicee (Cappella dei Principi and New Sacristy)
3. Mercato Centrale
4. Palazzo Medici Riccardi

Places to Eat

1. Da Garibaldi
2. La Bolognese
3. Trattoria La Gratella
4. Nerbone
5. Nannini
6. McDonald's

Accommodatior

1. Hotel Botticelli
2. Hotel Galileo
3. Hotel il Guelfo Bianco
4. Ostello Archi Rossi

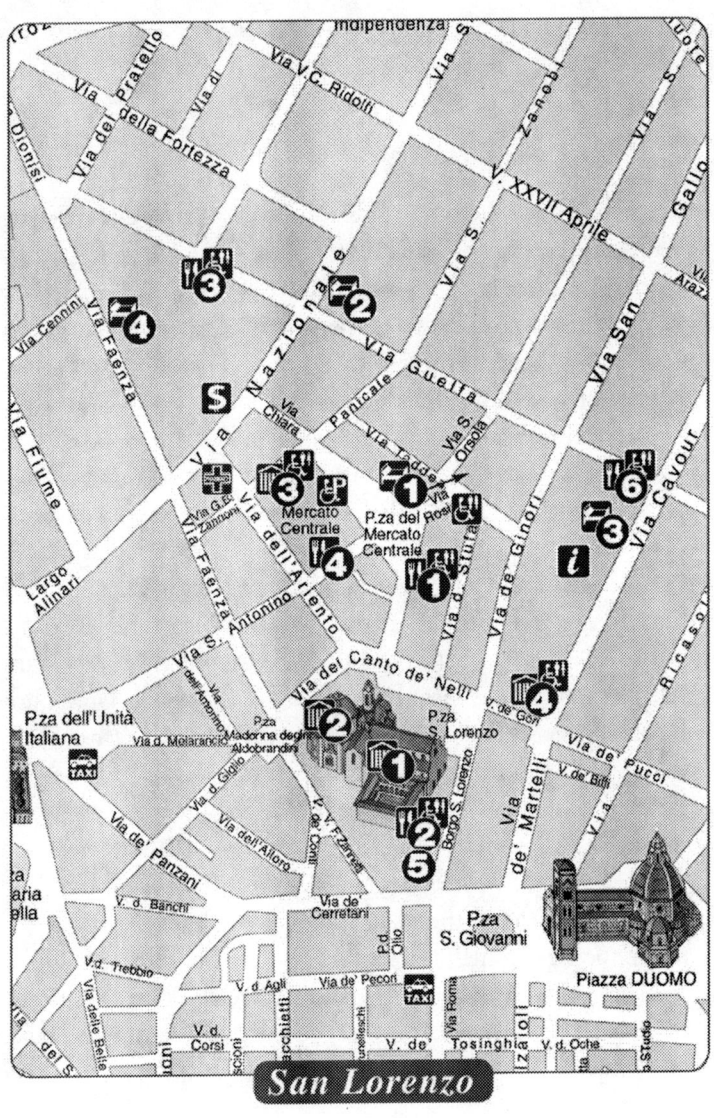

San Lorenzo

What to See

San Lorenzo (accessible with assistance)
Piazza San Lorenzo
Open: 10:00-17:00, Monday-Saturday; closed on Sundays and holidays
Information: 055 216 634
Admission: €2,50

Description: San Lorenzo, designed by Brunelleschi and constructed between 1419 and1469, is the first church to be built in the style of the early Florentine Renaissance with proportional planning, classical motifs, and a cool interior decorative scheme of gray-green stone and white plaster. Initially financed by the city, the project ran aground when the government encountered financial difficulties and was saved by a loan made by Cosimo de'Medici. In acknowledgment of his generosity, the Medici were allowed to display their coat of arms in the nave and over the crossing of the church and from that time San Lorenzo, to all effects, became their church. As the fame of the family grew, pieces were added on to the complex. The **Old Sacristy**, designed by Brunelleschi and built between 1421 and 1429, doubled as a private family burial chapel. The **Laurentian Library**, designed by Michelangelo, housed their impressive collection of Greek and Roman manuscripts. Medici Pope Leo X announced a competition in 1515 to complete the church facade. Although never built, the winning project by Michelangelo is known through the artist's model, now visible in the Casa Buonarroti. Michelangelo then began work on a new set of family tombs called the **New Sacristy** built inside the church directly opposite Brunelleschi's Old Sacristy. The ornate **Cappella dei Principi**, located behind the church's main altar, was built as a burial chapel for the sixteenth—and seventeenth-century members of the family.

Accessibility: Entrance—A stone ramp on the far left leads from the level of the piazza to the raised platform in front of the church.

There are two steps to the church entrance and ticket office. (First step—height: 13 centimeters [5 ¼ inches]; width: 146 centimeters [57 ½" inches]. Second step—10 centimeters [4 inches]. The door that leads into the church measures 88 centimeters [34 ½ inches] in width). The nave and transepts of the church are level. Two **lightweight, portable track ramps are available for use at the entrance and to enter Brunelleschi's Old Sacristy** (three steps). **The New Sacristy is not wheelchair accessible** (see *Cappelle Medicee* below).The **Laurentian Library** is located on the second floor and is **not wheelchair accessible,** but its exterior facade is visible from the courtyard. Entrance to the courtyard is through the door at the top of the ramp in front of the church. There is a high lip on threshold of the courtyard entrance; irregular stone pavement under the courtyard porticoes; two flights of steps up to the library.

Comments: The custodians of the church are very helpful. If needed, the two track ramps can easily be brought to the main entrance, although the first step is so wide that some manual wheelchair users with assistance can probably manage without them.

Cappelle Medicee (limited accessibility)
Piazza Madonna degli Aldobrandini
Tel: 055 2 88 02
Open: Tuesday-Saturday and the second and fourth Monday and first, third, and fifth Sunday of the month, 8:15-16:50; closed the first, third, and fifth Monday and the second and fourth Sunday of the month
Admission: €6,00

Description: The Cappelle Medicee complex begins, just inside the entrance, with a ground-floor crypt containing tombs; however, the most important members of the family are buried in the chapels upstairs. The seventeenth-century **Cappella dei Principi** with its walls and floor covered with multicolored *pietra dura* stone, much of it carved by Turkish slaves captured during naval skirmishes on the Mediterranean, holds the tombs of six Medici grand dukes including Cosimo I and his two sons: Francesco I and Ferdinando I. The more famous chapel by Michelangelo, also known as the **New Sacristy**, holds the tombs of the last two heirs of the fifteenth-century family line: Giuliano, Duke of Nemour, and Lorenzo, Duke of Urbino, undistinguished in their lifetime but immortalized in their death by the beautiful tombs designed by the artist. The more famous Lorenzo the Magnificent and Giuliano, his brother, killed in the Pazzi Conspiracy, are also buried in the chapel together in an unfinished tomb.

Accessibility: There is **no elevator.** Two flights of stairs (twenty-six steps) lead to the upstairs tombs. A **handheld stair-climbing device,** operated by museum personnel and capable of carrying manual wheelchairs, **is available to reach the *Cappella dei Principi.*** Michelangelo's New Sacristy **is not accessible** to wheelchairs and is located four steps down from the level of the Prince's Chapel through a passage too narrow for the handheld device to operate safely. There is **no wheelchair-accessible restroom.**

Mercato di San Lorenzo
Piazza del Mercato Centrale and surrounding streets
Open: Monday-Saturday, 7:00-14:00 (food market); 8:30-19:00 (outside, clothing and souvenir stalls)

Description: The street market is located in the area around the Church of San Lorenzo, stretching west to Via Nazionale and surrounding the central food market. Best approaches are either from Via Nazionale, taking Via dell'Ariento, or from Via Martelli/ Via Cavour, taking Via de'Gori. Stands sell everything from leather jackets, gloves, belts, and handbags to sweaters, shoes and socks, underwear, secondhand clothes, and souvenirs. The stands closer to the church and nearer Via Nazionale seem to cater more to tourists; those along the flanks of the food market, more to the locals.

The colorful central food market is located in a big nineteenth-century cast-iron building. Ground-floor stands sell meat and poultry, wild game, fish, bread, cheese, truffles, and pasta. Upstairs are the fruit, vegetable, and flower vendors. On the east side of the market is the lunch stand **Nerbone**, a market landmark most famous for its sandwiches (the Florentines go for the tripe), but with equally good assorted pasta, salad, and meat dishes.

Accessibility: The market is accessible by **two ramps**: one on the south side at Via dell'Ariento, 10 (entrance to the ramp is located between the second and third stands down from the corner of Via dell'Ariento and Via S. Antonino); the other, on the north side at Piazza del Mercato Centrale, 5. There are two **elevators**: one located inside the Via dell'Ariento entrance near the southwest corner; the other, outside next to the north ramp in Piazza del Mercato Centrale. There are two **wheelchair-accessible restrooms** on the southwest corner of the market: one is on the ground floor next to the stairs to the street; the other, upstairs next to the elevator. The ground-floor restroom is cleaner but small and suitable only for small wheelchairs. (Entering the restroom, the WC is located to the immediate right with a fixed grab bar on the right wall while space to transfer is from the left side near the door. The key to this restroom is kept at Signor Sacchetti's butcher stand opposite the elevator.) Although the restroom upstairs is larger, at the time of inspection for this guide, it was closed for repairs.

Comments: If you decide to have lunch at Nerbone's, there is a seating area opposite the food stall (step up: 12 centimeters [4 ¾ inches]). Since there is generally a lack of seats during the crowded lunch hour, many people just hang out and munch on their sandwiches next to the counter. There are several other less-famous places to eat with accessible seating beyond Nerbone heading towards the north entrance.

Palazzo Medici Riccardi (partial accessibility)
Via Cavour, 1 (wheelchair-accessible entrance) and 3
Tel: 055 276 0340
Open: 9:00-19:00; closed on Wednesday
Admission: € 4,00; free for people who are disabled and their companions

Description: Palazzo Medici Riccardi was built for the banker Cosimo il Vecchio in 1444 and remained the Medici family home until 1540 when Duke Cosimo I moved to the Palazzo Vecchio. In his design for the palace, the architect Michelozzo skillfully blended traditional elements of local medieval palace architecture with classical motifs, drawing inspiration from the Arch of Constantine in Rome for the heavy overhanging cornice. The Riccardi family bought the palace in the seventeenth century, enlarging the facade by seven bays, to include sumptuous rooms, some decorated by Luca Giordano, a leading Baroque artist.

Accessibility: Wheelchair-accessible entrance is through the main door into the palace courtyard. Guard on duty will open gate. Bookstore, elevator, and accessible restroom are through the door to the right of the main courtyard. The **wheelchair-accessible restroom** is located between the main courtyard and the *Corte dei Muli* (fixed grab bar to left of WC; retractable bar to right; space for right transfer; key is kept in the bookstore). Entrance to the ground-floor exhibition rooms is in the main courtyard to the left. Threshold lips are found at most doors in these rooms. To see the upstairs room decorated by Luca Giordano, take the elevator to the second floor (elevator door width: 76 ½ centimeters [30 inches]; cabin width: 108 centimeters [42 ½ inches]; cabin length: 88 centimeters [34 ¾ inches]), then the stair lift down one flight of stairs with handrail. At present, access to the *Cappella dei Magi* painted by Benozzo Gozzoli is by a four-flight grand staircase only (no handrail; sixty-five steps). The entrance into the chapel has one step: 10 centimeters (4 inches) up; 6 centimeters (2 ³/₈ inches) down.

Comments: Future plans include enlarging the elevator and creating wheelchair access to the Gozzoli Chapel.

San Marco

Tree-shaded Piazza San Marco teems with university students, tourists, and commuters. The administrative offices of the University of Florence are housed in the former grand ducal stables on the east side of the square. On the southeast corner the entrance to the **Accademia delle Belle Arti**, the city's art academy, is through the loggia once part of San Matteo, a fourteenth-century hospital. To the south is a string of restaurants, bars and cafés, and a major bus stop; to the west, a curious eighteenth-century palazzo built for the mistress of the Lorraine grand duke Pietro Leopoldo. Next door a long wall extends north towards the entrance to the Court of Appeals located in the former **Casino di San Marco**, built in the sixteenth century by the architect Buontalenti for Francesco I to house the laboratories in which the Medici duke conducted his experiments in alchemy. The Church and Convent of San Marco, which now houses the **Museo di San Marco**, dominate the north side of the square.

Other sights in the San Marco neighborhood are within short distance. The **Cenacolo di Sant'Apollonia** lies two blocks to the west of the square. To the north, down Via Cavour and just beyond the Court of Appeals, is the **Chiostro dello Scalzo**. Via La Pira, next to the university, leads towards the **Museo di Geologia e Paleotologia** and the **Botanical Gardens** known as the **Giardino dei Semplici**. Via C. Battisti to the east takes you into Piazza Santissima Annunziata with Brunelleschi's orphanage, the **Ospedale degli Innocenti**, and beyond the piazza, to the **Archaeological Museum**. Down Via Ricasoli and just past the Accademia delle Belle Arti loggia is the entrance to the **Galleria dell'Accademia**, now home to Michelangelo's *David.* The **Museo delle Pietre Dure** is just around the corner in Via Alfani. To get there, make a left after the little square in front of Florence's "Luigi Cherubini" Music Conservatory.

Mobility

Getting There

Wheelchair-accessible Bus 7 leaves from the RR station, making stops in Via Martelli (between Piazza San Giovanni and Palazzo Medici Riccardi) and in Piazza San Marco before going to Fiesole. On the return trip from Fiesole, the stop nearest to Piazza San Marco is in Via Cavour just before the piazza. There are two other stops in Via Cavour—the first, for Palazzo Medici Riccardi; the second, for Piazza San Giovanni—before arriving at the RR station.

Nonwheelchair-accessible electric Bus C leaves Piazza San Marco making stops in Piazza SS Annunziata, Sant'Ambrogio (produce market), and Santa Croce, before heading across the river to Piazza Santa Maria Sopr'Arno near the Ponte Vecchio. Return trip from Piazza Santa Maria Sopr'Arno takes you back across the river to Santa Croce, Piazza dei Ciompi (flea market), the Museo Archeologico, Piazza SS Annunziata, ending up in Piazza San Marco.

Getting Around

Most main streets have wide sidewalks with curb cuts including Via Cavour from Piazza San Marco south to Piazza del Duomo and north to Viale Matteotti, Via Giorgio La Pira north from Piazza San Marco towards the Giardino dei Semplici, Via XXVII Aprile from Piazza San Marco west to Piazza Indipendenza, Via Cesare Battisti east to Piazza SS Annunziata. The section of Via Ricasoli from Piazza San Marco to Via Alfani is a pedestrian zone. Irregular pavement and narrow sidewalks make Via Della Colonna (Archaeological Museum) and the bottom of Via de'Servi near the Duomo much less wheelchair friendly, and the going can sometimes be hazardous.

There is a **taxi stand** in Piazza San Marco.

Designated parking spaces are located on the east side of Piazza San Marco (two spaces), in front of the entrance to the Botanical Gardens in Via Micheli (one space), in Via San Gallo above Via XVII Aprile in front of the loggia on the right at n. 34A (two spaces), and in Piazza Brunelleschi. To enter this small piazza, turn right from Via de' Servi into Via del Castellaccio.

Driving is restricted throughout this area of town which is part of the limited traffic zone (ZTL). See "Driving Around" in the chapter on "Transportation" for further explanation.

What the Neighborhood Has to Offer

This neighborhood has few places to eat which are easily accessible. **Pugi** (open Monday-Saturday), a take-out bakery reputed by many to have the best pizza and *schiacciata* in town, is on the south side of Piazza San Marco at no. 10. Heading south of the piazza towards the Duomo down Via Cavour, there is a **McDonald's** on the corner of Via Guelfa with a level entrance and wheelchair-accessible restroom. A number of places to eat are found to the west of the piazza. **Nabucco**, a wine bar across from the *Cenacolo di Sant'Apollonia*, has a step at the main entrance and a locked, wheelchair-accessible entrance around the corner which is opened on request. **Semidivino** (Via S. Gallo 22/r), a restaurant/wine bar with outside seating, serves Tuscan specialties (accessible restroom; one step at entrance). One block north of Via XVII Aprile in Via delle Ruote, 30/r **Il Vegetariano**, an informal and often crowded, vegetarian, cafeteria-style restaurant, has been popular with the Florentines since the 1970s (one step at entrance; steep ramp to back rooms; wheelchair-accessible restroom without grab bars).

Near the Museo delle Pietre Dure in Via Alfani,70/r, near the corner of Via de'Servi, is a popular and very crowded place called

Buffet Freddo (level entrance; open 9:00-16:30, closed on Sundays) serving delicious, typical, straightforward Florentine food which you order at the counter and have brought to one of the small tables. To avoid the rush, and sometimes just to get in the door, avoid going between 12:30 and 14:00.

If you're coming from or going to the Duomo in Via de'Servi, 40/r, **Caffè Fiorino**, a small bar, serves sandwiches and has a decent, accessible restroom.

Accessibility Checklist

The following list contains information on various places which are accessible to wheelchairs.

Accommodations

- Hotel Carolus
- Hotel de la Pace
- Hotel Orto de'Medici
- Residence San Gallo

Places to Eat

- Buffet Freddo
- Caffè Fiorino
- Il Vegetariano
  One step at entrance. Steep internal ramp. Self-service.
- McDonald's in Via Cavour
- Nabucco
  The wheelchair-accessible entrance around the corner in Via Santa Reparata is kept locked and is opened on request. There is one step at the main entrance.
- Semidivino
  One high step at entrance. Outside seating. Accessible restroom.

Accessible Restrooms

- Galleria dell'Accademia
- Giardino dei Semplici (Botanical Gardens)
  Located inside the gardens.
- Hotel Carolus
  There is an accessible restroom on the ground floor near the bar to the right of the reception desk. WC has fixed grab bar on right wall; transfer space on left.
- Museo Archeologico
- Museo di San Marco
  One step at entrance to museum.
- Museo dell'Opificio delle Pietre Dure
  One step or small platform lift to restroom.
- Caffè Fiorino
- Il Vegetariano
  One step at entrance. Steep internal ramp. Restroom without grab bars.
- McDonald's
- Nabucco
  You have to pass through swinging doors to reach the accessible restroom. Suitable only for smaller wheelchairs.
- Semidivino
  One step at entrance.

Pharmacies

- Farmacia Brizio Mazzei
  Via XXVII Aprile, 23/r
  Tel: 055 211 787
  Level entrance with automatic door. Also sells homeopathic medicines.

San Marco

Monuments

1. Church of San Marco
2. Museum of San Marco
3. Cenacolo of Sant'Apollonia
4. Giardino dei Semplici (Botanical Gardens)
5. Museo di Geologia e Paleontologia
6. Galleria dell'Accademia
7. Opificio delle Pietre Dure
8. Church of SS. Annunziata
9. Ospedale degli Innocenti
10. Archeological Museum

Places to Eat

1. Buffet Freddo
2. Café Fiorino
3. Il Vegetariano
4. McDonald's
5. Nabucco
6. Semidivino

Accommodations

1. Hotel Carolus
2. Hotel de la Pace
3. Hotel Orto de'Medici
4. Residence San Gallo

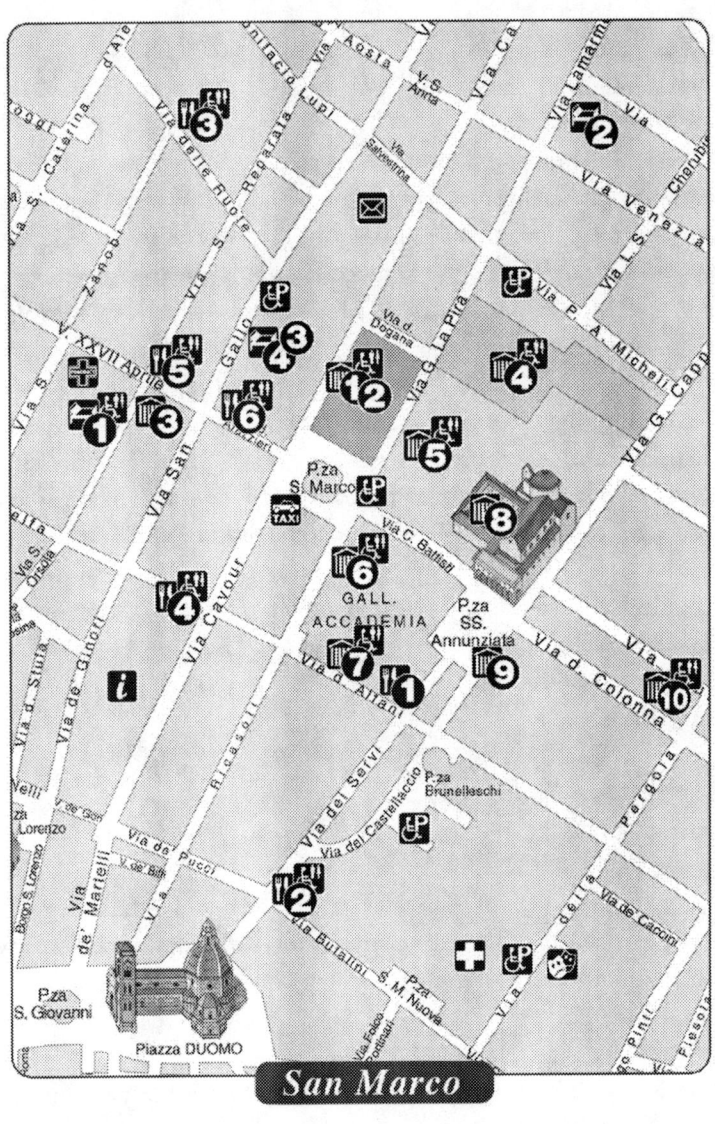

San Marco

What to See

San Marco (not accessible to wheelchairs)
Piazza San Marco
Open: 8:30-12:00; 16:00-18:00; Sunday, 16:00-18:00
Admission: Free

Description: In 1437 Cosimo il Vecchio de'Medici commissioned the architect Michelozzo for the construction of the Dominican Church and Convent of San Marco. The best things to see, the frescoes and altarpieces by Fra Angelico, are in the former convent, now a museum, next door. The church is somewhat of a disappointment from its nondescript eighteenth-century facade to its rather anonymous interior aside from the beautiful Chapel of Sant'Antonino, dedicated to the Dominican bishop and founder of the convent and church. His chapel, designed by Giambologna, has early seventeenth-century frescoes in the dome by Poccetti and a beautiful *Christ in Limbo* by Alessandro Allori on the altar (1588).

Accessibility: There are two steps to the podium in front of the church. The steps are lower from the left sidewalk. Once inside, everything is on one level with a small ramp to enter the Chapel of Sant'Antonino.

Museo di San Marco (accessible with assistance)
Piazza San Marco, 1
Tel: 055 238 8608
Open: Monday-Friday, 8:15-13:50; Saturday, 8:15-18:50; Sunday, 8:15-19:00; closed on first, third, fifth Sunday and second and fourth Monday of each month
Admission: €6,00

Description: The highlights of this museum are the paintings by Fra Angelico, the Dominican friar from nearby Fiesole, who was commissioned around the mid-fifteenth century for the decorations of the new church and convent. His brightly colored decorative *Pala di San Marco* for the high altar clearly expressed the

Dominicans' debt to the Medici for their financial support in the construction of the church. Medici patron saints Cosmas and Damian are seen kneeling on a Turkish carpet whose perspective lines create a deep spatial setting for the Christ child and the enthroned Madonna surrounded by angels and saints. On the left Cosimo de' Medici appears in the guise of the kneeling Saint Cosmas. St. John the Baptist (second standing figure from the left) is probably a portrait of his father, Giovanni, and St. Lawrence, next to him, of his brother Lorenzo who died in 1440, the year the painting was completed. Red balls decorate the gold-colored edge of the carpet making a clear reference to the Medici family coat of arms. Upstairs, the "Blessed" Angelico and his assistants painted each of the austere friars' cells with a contemplative and powerful image reflecting the Dominican's belief of mankind's redemption through Christ. Cosimo was given a special corner cell near the library built for him by Michelozzo to hold his collection of antique manuscripts. Savonarola's cell is located at the opposite end of the corridor.

Accessibility: There is a step down at the entrance to the ticket office (17 centimeters [6 ¾ inches]). Short ramps are located throughout the ground-floor rooms; the one leading into the *Sala Capitolare* is particularly steep. The **wheelchair-accessible route** to see Ghirlandaio's *Last Supper* in the refectory is through the *Sala del Lavabo* located off the far-right corner of the main courtyard. Turn left from the Sala del Lavabo into a small courtyard. In the courtyard, take the door to the left which brings you into the corridor leading to the refectory and bookstore.

An **accessible restroom** is located on the right in the small courtyard (WC 54 centimeters [21 ¼ inches] high, sits on pedestal base; grab bars to right and rear; space for left transfer).

To view Michelozzo's library and the monk's cells decorated by Fra Angelico upstairs, continue straight through the small courtyard into a third courtyard for the **stair lift** (71 centimeters [28 inches] wide; 86 centimeters [33 ⁷/₈ inches] long; capacity: 120 kilograms [264 pounds]). You will exit from the stair lift directly into Michelozzo's library. The entire second floor is wheelchair accessible except for the cells of Cosimo de'Medici (six steps) and Savonarola (three steps).

There are high lips at some ground-floor doorway thresholds. The staircase to the second floor has three steep flights of stairs (forty-two steps) with handrails. **No elevator**. Some scattered seating. Labeling of works of art is in Italian only. **Eleven steps lead to the exit at rear of museum. Wheelchairs exit is back through the entrance at Piazza San Marco.**

Comments: The stair lift to the second floor is located on an exterior staircase and cannot be operated when it is raining. A manual wheelchair has been requested by the museum for use of visitors. Call the number given above for latest information.

Cenacolo di Sant'Apollonia (accessible with assistance)
Via XXVII Aprile, 1 (west of Piazza San Marco)
Tel: 055 238 8607
Open: 8:30-13:50 every day except the second and fourth Monday and the first, third, and fifth Sunday of every month
Admission: Free

Description: The explosive pattern in the marble panel above the heads of St. Peter, Judas, and Christ dramatically unites themes of denial, betrayal, and salvation in Andrea del Castagno's *Last Supper* (1447). Only the cloistered Benedictine nuns for whom it was painted were allowed to view it until the convent was expropriated by the Kingdom of Italy in the nineteenth century.

Accessibility: Sidewalks in this neighborhood have curb cuts. Entrance has one step (8 centimeters [3 1/8 inches]) through double doors. Each door (66 centimeters [26 inches]) can be opened. Short ramp into refectory. Seating. **No accessible restroom.**

Comments: On the same side of the street towards Piazza Indipendenza, you'll find an accessible restroom in the lobby of the nearby Hotel Carolus.

Chiostro dello Scalzo (accessible with assistance)
Via Cavour, 69 (north of Piazza San Marco)
Open: 8:15-13:50, Monday, Thursday, and Saturday
Admission: Free

Description: This is a small but magnificent sixteenth-century courtyard painted in *grisaille* or monochrome fresco between 1511 and 1526 by Andrea del Sarto, with the help of Franciabigio, for the Confraternity of the Disciples of Saint John the Baptist whose duties included burying condemned prisoners as emphasized by the skull-and-crossbones motif which appear in the capital bases and in some of the painted decoration. The four cardinal virtues and scenes from the life of Florence's patron saint, John the Baptist, are depicted and demonstrate the development of del Sarto's style from the still-timid *Baptism of Christ* of 1509/1510 to the full-blown High Renaissance *Baptism of the Multitudes* of 1517 where several of the foreground figures were inspired by Michelangelo's famous and now lost fresco of the *Battle of Cascina* once in the Palazzo Vecchio.

Accessibility: Step at threshold is 2.5 centimeters (1 inch) up; 5 centimeters (2 inches) down. Entrance is through two sets of double wooden doors, both swing inwards. Short ramp into vestibule. The small *chiostro* or courtyard presents no obstacles. Seating. Written descriptions are in Italian only. **No accessible restroom.**

Comments: Nearest accessible restroom is in the San Marco Museum (closed the second and fourth Monday of the month).

Giardino dei Semplici (accessible with assistance)
Via Micheli, 3 (north of Piazza San Marco)
Tel: 055 275 7402
Open: Monday-Friday, 9:00-13:00
Admission: €3,00; €1,50 for students six to fourteen years old. Free for children under six, adults over sixty-five, and for people who are disabled.

Description: The Giardino dei Semplici (herb garden) was founded in 1550 by Cosimo dei Medici and is one of the oldest botanical gardens in the world. The over 5,500 different specimens in the collection are cultivated outdoors or in greenhouses and include carnivorous plants, exotic orchids, cork and fig trees, and a medicinal flower bed.

Accessibility: There is a **ramp down to the garden level** beyond the ticket counter and an **accessible restroom** (fixed grab bars on left; room for right transfer) in the garden. Paths have loose gravel and firmly packed dirt surfaces. Seating is mostly found in the central area around the fountain. Many greenhouses are closed to the public, and most are unaccessible to wheelchairs. One designated parking space is located in front of the entrance.

Comments: This is a cool, summertime alternative to crowded museums. A free pamphlet with map of the garden and a detailed guide in English for sale are available at the ticket counter. Plants are identified with their botanical Latin names.

Museo di Geologia e Paleontologia
Via La Pira, 4 (north of Piazza San Marco)
Tel: 055 275 7536
Open: Tuesday-Saturday, 9:00-13:00; Tuesday afternoon, 14:00-17:00; closed on Sunday and Monday
Admission: €4,00; €2,00 for children six to eighteen years old

Description: Part of the University of Florence, this museum contains an important collection of fossils, traces the evolution of the horse, and displays some impressive elephant skeletons found in the Valdarno valley south of Florence. VIVAT conducts tactile tours by appointment. Labeling of exhibits is in Italian.

Accessibility: There is a ramp at the entrance and accessible WC (grab bars and space for left transfer). For information on tactile tours see "Museums, Music, Movies, and Sports."

Galleria dell'Accademia
Via Ricasoli, 58 and 60 (wheelchair-accessible entrance)
Tel: 055 238 8609
Open: Tuesday-Sunday, 8:15-18:50; closed on Monday
Admission: €6,50

Description: Michelangelo's *David,* carved to decorate one of the high buttresses of the Duomo, and the *Slaves,* commissioned for Pope Julius II's tomb in St. Peter's in Rome, need no introduction. The rest of the works exhibited in the galleries are plaster casts and paintings from the thirteenth to sixteenth centuries gathered for purposes of study for the students of Florence's art academy or *Accademia* originally founded under the Medici in 1563. Some important works include Giambologna's full-scale plaster model of the *Rape of the Sabine Women* prepared for execution of the marble statue now under the Loggia dei Lanzi; the *Adimari Cassone,* a fourteenth-century painted wedding chest with a view of the Baptistery, and several *Madonnas* attributed to Botticelli. Of special interest is a superb collection of antique musical instruments, some commissioned by the Medici, which has been recently put on display in the ground-floor rooms located to the right just inside the entrance to the first gallery.

Accessibility: One wheelchair is available. Request from one of the museum personnel in the main entrance hall. From the wheelchair entrance, turn right into the main entrance hall for access to the galleries. The entire ground floor is accessible; a ramp leads to the collection of plaster casts by the eighteenth-century sculptor Lorenzo Bartolini. The **accessible restroom,** located on the ground floor, is reached by turning left at the *David,* going left through the Italian primitive rooms, around the glassed-in courtyard and turning right. (WC height: 52 centimeters [20 ½ inches]; grab bars to right and rear.) More restrooms (not accessible) are located downstairs near the gallery exit. An **elevator** to the second floor is located opposite the restroom. On the upper floor, fourteen steps lead to the first gallery; then seven steps to the level of the remaining galleries. Two stair lifts, operated by the museum guards, provide access to these galleries for wheelchair users. First stair lift—max weight: 150 kilograms (330 pounds); length: 84 centimeters (33 inches). Second stair lift—max weight: 130 kilograms (286 pounds); length 80 centimeters (31 ½ inches).

Comments: Unless you are passionately interested in large fifteenth-century altarpieces, the best things to see are on the ground floor. The Accademia probably has one of Florence's original, accessible restrooms, and the pedestal base, built under the WC to raise its height, could create a problem in transferring for some people.

Museo dell'Opificio delle Pietre Dure
Via Alfani, 78
Tel: 055 265 111
Open: Monday-Saturday, 8:15-14:00; Thursday, 8:15-19:00; closed on Sundays and holidays
Admission: €2,00

Description: Originally the *Opificio* was a workshop opened by Ferdinando I de'Medici in 1588 for the carving of semiprecious stones set in mosaic used to decorate the floor, walls, and altars of the new family mausoleum in San Lorenzo, the Chapel of the Princes. Today it is a delightful small museum. The ground floor contains objects and furniture, many pieces once belonging to the Medici. Examples of semiprecious stones and the instruments used to carve them are displayed on the balcony upstairs.

Accessibility: Ingenious **platform lift** rises out of the pavement (80 centimeters by 137 centimeters [31 ½ inches by 54 inches]) to overcome the one step to ticket office, bookstore, and **accessible restroom** (WC 53 centimeters [21 inches]; grab bars to right and rear; left transfer) and to the museum. There is a **stair lift** inside the museum to the upstairs balcony (67 centimeters [26 ³/8 inches] wide; 75 centimeters [29 ½ inches] long; capacity: 150 kilograms

[330 pounds]). The last room on the ground floor has one step down (18 centimeters [just over 7 inches]), then one step at the exit door (20 centimeters [7 $^7/8$ inches]). To avoid these steps, retrace your path to the entrance. Scattered seating is available. Labeling is in Italian only.

Comments: This charming, off-the-beaten-path, very accessible museum offers a peaceful interlude to the crowds around the corner at the Accademia.

Santissima Annunziata (atrium accessible; assistance advised for entering the church)
Piazza SS Annunziata
Tel: 055 266 181
Open: 7:30-12:30; 16:00-18:30
Admission: Free

Description: There are two important fresco cycles in the atrium. The one on the right depicts the life of the Virgin and was painted between 1511 and 1517 by the Mannerist artists Andrea del Sarto (*Voyage of the Magi* and *Birth of the Virgin*), Franciabigio (*Marriage of the Virgin*), Pontormo (*Visitation*), and Rosso il Fiorentino (*Assumption*) with an earlier *Nativity* by Alessio Baldovinetti (1460-1462) painted on the wall directly behind the image of the famous *Annunciation* inside the church. The other cycle by del Sarto and Cosimo Rosselli depicts the life of San Filippo Benizzi, one of the founders in 1234 of the "Servants of Mary," the Servite order for whom the church and convent were originally built. The entire complex was rebuilt by Michelozzo, architect of nearby San Marco around 1444-1455. Inside the church to the left of the main entrance is the altar dedicated to the Virgin or "la Santissima Annunziata" to whom the church is dedicated. This church has always had great importance for the Florentines, not only for the miraculous image of the Annunciation on the altar which according to legend was begun by a monk and finished by an angel, but also because, until the seventeenth-century reform by Grand Duke Pietro

Leopoldo, the Florentine calendar began the new year on March 25, feast day of the Annunciation.

Accessibility: A **sidewalk ramp to porch level** is located to the left of the church in Via Cesare Battisti, followed by a **ramp** on the left inside the entrance to the atrium. Heavy, swinging double doors lead into church proper (each 70 centimeters [27 ½ inches] wide) with threshold lip of 2.5 centimeters (1 inch). The nave and transepts are barrier free with two steps to the side chapels which are also visible from the floor level. There are five steps up and one step down into the rotonda behind the main altar.

Comments: The best things to see, the frescoes in the atrium and the two frescoes by Andrea del Castagno in the church interior, are easily visible. Ask the sacristan to uncover Castagno's *St. Julian* fresco (1455) hidden behind a Baroque painting on hinges in the first chapel to the left. In the following chapel is Castagno's *Trinity* (1454-1455) with St. Jerome and Two Maries.

Museo dello Spedale degli Innocenti (partial accessibility)
Piazza SS Annunziata
Tel: 055 249 1708
Open: Every day except Wednesday, 8:30-14:00
Admission: €2,60

Description: Filippo Brunelleschi, architect of the cathedral cupola visible from the piazza and of the churches of San Lorenzo and Santo Spirito, made his Renaissance architectural debut in 1419 with the design of the **Ospedale degli Innocenti**, a foundling hospital, identified by the della Robbia ceramic swaddling wrapped infants appearing on the facade. The use of harmonic proportions and the simple, repetitive semicircular arches carried on Corinthian columns marked a revolutionary return to classical language, and the building was recognized as a landmark in the architect's lifetime. Today the *ospedale* houses a recreation center for children, a public health clinic, a temporary home for unwed mothers and, upstairs, a painting gallery.

Accessibility: The painting gallery, located on the top floor, is reached by three steep flights of stairs with handrail (**no elevator**). Wheelchair-accessible entrance to view the two courtyards designed by Brunelleschi is located at Piazza SS Annunziata, 13. Just inside this door a steep ramp with a no-skid surface leads to the courtyard level. **No accessible restroom.**

Comments: While the painting gallery is off limits for many, some may not want to miss a chance to get a backstage view of this milestone in Renaissance architecture. The orphans lived in the rooms around the first and smallest of the two courtyards. Go to the end of this courtyard and turn left for the larger courtyard which is decorated with frescoed symbols: the door represented the silk guild who financed the construction. Outside, at one end of the main porch, steps lead up to a window, once with a turntable behind it, where the unwanted children were left. You do not have to pay to see the courtyards or the porch which can be partially viewed through the main door (steps).

Museo Archeologico (accessible with assistance)
Via della Colonna, 38
Tel: 055 235 750
Open: Monday, 14:00-19:00; Tuesday and Thursday, 8:30-19:00; Wednesday, Friday, Saturday, and Sunday, 8:30-14:00
Admission: €4,00

Description: The original nucleus of objects in this museum, which was founded in 1870, belonged to fifteenth-century Medici: Cosimo il Vecchio and his grandson, Lorenzo the Magnificent, with their collection of antique gems, now displayed in the Medici corridor, and sculptures, including the magnificent Hellenistic bronze horse head, once part of a fountain in the Medici family palace. In the sixteenth century, Duke Cosimo I expanded the family collection with important Etruscan finds: the *Chimera*, the *Minerva*, and the *Orator* (*L'Arringatore*) found during excavations in southern Tuscany and Umbria. Enlarged with nineteenth-century acquisitions, including the nucleus of the Egyptian art collection, and with important discoveries from the excavations of Etruscan tombs, such as the famous Greek Attic *François* vase found in 1845 near Chiusi, the collection now ranks as one of the most important in Italy.

Accessibility: The museum located on the second and third floors is reached by staircase or, accompanied by museum personnel, by large **elevator.** On the second floor (1° *piano*) wheelchair access to the Etruscan rooms overlooking the courtyard is by **stair lift** (width: 71.5 centimeters [28 ¼ inches]; length: 92 centimeters [36 ¼ inches]; capacity: 150 kilograms [330 pounds]). Wheelchair access to the Medici Corridor with its collection of Medici gems is by **stair lift** (width: 65 centimeters [25 ½ inches]; length: 86 centimeters [33 ⁷/₈ inches]; capacity: 150 kilograms [330 pounds]). The third floor (2° *piano*) presents no obstacles. There is a **wheelchair-accessible restroom** on the ground floor in an area reserved for museum personnel (grab bar on left; room for right transfer). The third-floor restrooms are not accessible.

Comments: Wheelchair users will have to rely on the very courteous museum personnel for their visit. Guided tours are given in the garden on Saturday morning. Call museum for information.

Santa Croce

Traditionally a working-class neighborhood, during the Middle Ages and Renaissance, Santa Croce was populated by laborers from the cloth industry that formed the backbone of the city's wealth. Great drying sheds lined the banks of the Arno which supplied the water essential for washing and rinsing while dying workshops were crammed into nearby **Corso dei Tintori**, the "street of the dyers." So renowned was the industry that cloth was even sent from distant England and France to be dyed with the deep, rich colors that made Florentine textiles famous throughout Europe. When the new Franciscan order moved into town, it chose to settle in this humble neighborhood and minister to its poor, building the great **Church and Convent of Santa Croce**.

Today a new industry dominates Santa Croce: tourist shops and souvenir stalls now line the edges of the square where the Franciscans once preached to the underpaid workers. To find a taste of the real Florence, you need to wander through the side streets leading off the square over towards **Piazza dei Ciompi**, named after the workers revolt in the fourteenth century, or to the city market at **Sant'Ambrogio**.

Mobility

Getting There

Wheelchair-accessible **Bus 23** (direction: "Sorgane"), after leaving the station and passing by the Duomo, stops behind the Uffizi ("Galleria degli Uffizi") before crossing the river and heading towards Piazza Ferrucci. Return trip (direction "Zona Industriale") passes through Piazza Ferrucci, crossing the river at Ponte alle Grazie before making a stop in Via Verdi near Piazza Santa Croce, continuing on to Piazza Santa Maria Nuova (Museo di Firenze com'era) and the Duomo before returning to the station.

Electric Bus A (direction: "Beccaria"), not accessible to wheelchairs, leaves from the station making stops in Piazza Santa Maria Novella, next to the Church of Santa Trinita, in Via de'Pecori (Piazza del Duomo), Orsanmichele near Piazza della Repubblica, Via Ghibellina (Museo Bargello), Piazza dei Ciompi (flea market), and Borgo la Croce (Mercato di Sant'Ambrogio). Return trip stops (direction "Stazione") include Via dell'Agnolo (Mercato di Sant'Ambrogio*)*, Via Condotta (Piazza della Signoria), Via Strozzi (Piazza della Repubblica), Santa Maria Novella, and the station.

Electric Bus C (direction: "Santa Maria Sopr'Arno"), not accessible to wheelchairs, makes the following stops: Canto alla Pace (Mercato di Sant'Ambrogio), Magliabechi (Santa Croce) before heading across the Arno. Return trip (direction: "San Marco") leaves from Piazza S. Maria Sopr'Arno near the Ponte Vecchio passing by Piazza Santa Croce, Piazza dei Ciompi (flea market), and Sant'Ambrogio before heading towards Piazza SS Annunziata and Piazza San Marco.

Getting Around

Piazza Santa Croce is a leisurely ten or fifteen minutes from Piazza della Signoria either down the direct route of Borgo dei Greci which is limited to pedestrian traffic or down Via de'Neri, then Borgo Santa Croce into the piazza.

The following streets are pedestrian zones: Borgo dei Greci, Piazza Santa Croce, Via Pietrapiana towards Sant'Ambrogio, and Borgo La Croce from the market area to Piazza Beccaria. Via de'Neri has recently been repaved. Via A. Magliabechi between Piazza Santa Croce and Corso dei Tintori, Corso dei Tintori, Via de'Benci, and its continuation Via Verdi have sidewalks with curb cuts. The south side of Piazza Santa Croce where the tourist stands are set up is recommended for wheelchair users. The pavement in the rest of the piazza is extremely bumpy and irregular.

Taxi stands are located at the top of Piazza Santa Croce near Via Verdi and in Piazza Beccaria near the Credito Italiano bank.

Designated parking spaces are found near Piazza Santa Croce in Via A. Magliabechi on the right as you head towards Corso dei Tintori and in Via Verdi near the corner of Via Ghibellina on the left behind the Teatro Verdi. Public parking lots are located on the east side of the *Mercato di Sant'Ambrogio* and in Viale Giovine Italia (as you head towards the river on the right just beyond Via dell'Agnolo). A large underground parking lot is presently under construction near Piazza Beccaria. By tacit agreement, disability parking permit holders who have received permission to enter the ZTL are allowed to park inside the chained-off area at the top of Piazza Santa Croce near Via Verdi and only in the space not reserved for taxis, even though this parking area is not marked.

Viale Giovine Italia is open to normal traffic and the parking lot at the Mercato di Sant'Ambrogio can be accessed from Via dell'Agnolo. **However, you will need permission to drive in other parts of this neighborhood which is part of the ZTL (Limited Traffic Zone).** See the chapter on "Transportation" for details.

What the Neighborhood Has to Offer

A flea market chock full of "antique" bric-a-brac, a nineteenth-century cast-iron building housing a produce market, a main post office, and one of the best ice-cream shops in the city can be found around Santa Croce. The *gelateria* **Vivoli** (Via Isola delle Stinche, 7/r; closed on Monday; no accessible restroom) is a Florentine institution offering some of the best ice cream in the city. A number of *ristoranti, trattorie,* and cafés offer various wheelchair-accessible alternatives for eating: in the small piazza at the end of Borgo degli Albizzi, the **Ristorante/Pizzeria I Ghibellini** (Piazza S Pier Maggiore, 8/10; closed on Wednesday; one step at entrance; accessible restroom); near Piazza Santa Croce: **Ristorante Finisterrae** (Piazza Santa Croce, 12; accessible restroom). Next to the Mercato di

Sant'Ambrogio is the **Ristorante Cibreo** (Via A. del Verocchio, 8/r; closed Sunday-Monday; accessible restroom, one step at entrance). On the corner of Via de' Neri is the **Trattoria da Benvenuto** (Via della Mosca, 16/r; closed on Sunday; short ramp at entrance; accessible restroom without grab bars).

A **tourist information office** is located near Piazza Santa Croce in Borgo Santa Croce, 29/r.

Public, accessible restrooms are located in Borgo Santa Croce, 29/r, and in Via Filippina, corner Via Borgognona, located between Palazzo Vecchio and Piazza Santa Croce. The **post office** at the end of Via Verdi (accessible entrance is in Via Pietrapiana, 53) offers full service and is accessible to wheelchair users. Open Monday-Friday, 8:15-19:00, and Saturday, 8:15-12:30.

Accessibility Checklist

The following list contains information on various places which are accessible to wheelchairs.

Accomodations

- Hotel Bernini
- Hotel Rita Major

Places to Eat

- Goal Bar
  Light lunch
- Gusto Leo
- La Loggia degli Albizzi
  Sidewalk curb and steep ramp at entrance.
- Ristorante Cibreo
  One step at entrance.
- Ristorante Finisterrae
- Ristorante/Pizzeria I Ghibellini

One step at entrance.
- Trattoria da Benvenuto
- Trattoria Dante
No accessible restroom.

Accessible Restrooms

- Goal Bar
  Door swings in and opens to a maximum of 76 centimeters (30 inches). Transfer from right side of WC. Retractable grab bar on right only.
- Gusto Leo
  Fixed grab bar to right, retractable bar to left of WC (51 centimeters [20 inches] high).
- La Loggia degli Albizzi
  Fixed grab bar on wall to right, transfer space to left of WC. The position of the grab bar is slightly ahead of the WC.
- Ristorante Cibreo
  One step at entrance.
- Ristorante Finisterrae
- Ristorante/Pizzeria I Ghibellini
  One step at entrance.
- Trattoria da Benvenuto
  No grab bars.
- Museo del Bargello
  Stair lift to entrance of restroom.
- Museo di Antropologia e Etnologia
  Restroom is located to the left of the courtyard.
- Borgo Santa Croce 29/r
  Open: 10:00-18:00; summer, 9:00-19:00. Cost: €0,60
  Fixed grab bar to left, retractable grab bar and transfer space to right of WC.
- Via Filippina corner Via Borgognona
  Open: 9:00-19:00; summer, 9:00-19:00. Cost: €0,60

Internet Points

- Internet Train
  Borgo La Croce, 33/r
  Tel: 055 234 7852
  Open seven days a week until midnight. Monday-Saturday at 10:00; Sunday at 11:00. Level entrance from sidewalk. Sidewalk curb: 12 centimeters (4 ¾ inches).

- Internet Train
  Via de'Benci 36/r
  Tel: 055 263 8555
  Open seven days a week until 1:00 p.m. Monday-Friday at 9:00; Saturday at 10:00; Sunday at noon. Level entrance from sidewalk.

Banks

- Cassa di Risparmio, Agenzia 17
  Via Martiri del Popolo, 39/r (near Piazza dei Ciompi)
  Tel: 055 240 751
  Ring bell to enter. Three-centimeter (1 ¼-inch) lip at threshold.
- UniCredit
  Via G.Carducci, 2/r (near Piazza Sant'Ambrogio)
  Tel: 055 247 7638
  Ring bell to enter.
- Monte dei Paschi di Siena
  Via G Carducci, 11/r
  Ring bell to enter.
- Banca Nazionale di Lavoro
  Via Verdi, 18 (corner Via Ghibellina)
  Tel: 055 244 851
  Ring bell at foot of short entrance ramp.

- Credito Italiano
  Viale Giovine Italia, 15/r (corner Piazza Beccaria)
  Tel: 055 234 3658
  Ring bell to enter.
- Monte dei Paschi di Siena
  Piazza Beccaria, 5
  Tel: 055 241 073
  Ring bell to enter.

Santa Croce

Monuments

1. Casa Buonarroti
2. Mercato delle Pulci
3. Mercato di Sant'Ambrogio
4. Bargello Museum
5. Museo di Antropologia
6. Museo di Firenze com'era
7. Horne Museum
8. Church of Santa Croce and Museum
9. Church of Sant'Ambrogio
10. Synagogue and Museum

Places to Eat

1. Goal Bar
2. Trattoria Da Benvenuto
3. Gusto Leo
4. La Loggia degli Albizzi
5. Trattoria Dante
6. Ristorante Finisterrae
7. Ristorante/Pizzeria I Ghibellini
8. Trattoria Accadi
9. Ristorante Nonna Papera
10. Ristorante Cibreo
11. Da Rocco

Accommodations

1. Hotel Bernini
2. Hotel Rita Major

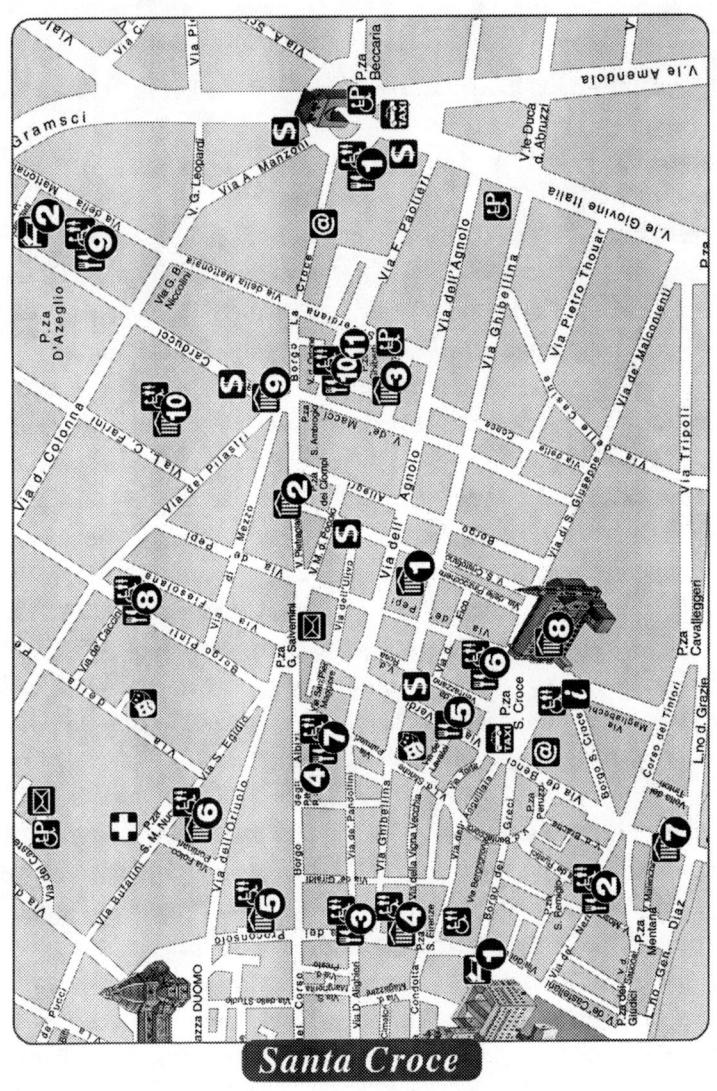

Santa Croce

What to See

Casa Buonarroti (conditioned accessibility and only with assistance)
Via Ghibellina, 70
Tel: 055 241 752
Open: Monday, Wednesday-Sunday, 9:30-14:00; closed on
Tuesday
Admission: €6,50

Description: Although Michelangelo once lived in a modest house
on this property, this small palace, known as Casa Buonarroti, was
built by his great nephew as tribute to the fame that the artist
brought to the Buonarroti family. Today a small museum, it holds
some important examples of Michelangelo's earliest works including
the *Battle of the Centaurs,* a marble relief panel he carved when
only fifteen years old, a piece which already embodied certain
themes developed around the nude male torso that were to recur
in works throughout the artist's career. The huge wooden
presentation model of San Lorenzo was the winning design in the
competition for the church facade that was never built. The
museum's intimate small rooms, some furnished and one decorated
with paintings to celebrate important events in Michelangelo's
lifetime, offer the chance to see a unique example of a domestic
seventeenth-century Florentine interior.

Accessibility: Conditioned accessibility is created by the two steps
at the entrance and the small size of the elevator. Entrance involves
one step at front door (15 centimeters [6 inches]), followed by one
step from the ticket office into the museum (17 centimeters [6 ¾
inches]). The bookshop, a courtyard, and three exhibition rooms
containing Etruscan and Roman artifacts, some art collected by
Michelangelo's descendants, and some derivative works by followers
of the artist, are located on the ground floor. The bulk of the
collection is upstairs and is reached by the main staircase (thirty
steps with handrail) or by elevator (door width: 55 centimeters
[21 ⅝ inches]; cabin length: 98 centimeters [38 ⅝ inches]; cabin
width: 89 centimeters [35 inches]).

Upstairs galleries are all on one level except for the *galleria* which has steep short ramps leading to a slightly raised platform which has been constructed to protect the terracotta flooring. The right-hand doors into the *galleria* and from the *galleria* into the successive rooms have narrower openings (70 centimeters [27 ½ inches]). There are slight lips on some door thresholds. The drawings exhibited in glass cases are too high to be seen from the level of a wheelchair. Scattered seating is found in the courtyard and in some upstairs galleries. Eight steps down from the upper floor or eighteen steps up from the courtyard lead to a mezzanine level where some small models and uninteresting plaster casts after Michelangelo's works are exhibited. Restrooms are off the upstairs galleries, but there is **no accessible restroom.**

Mercato delle Pulci (Flea Market)
Piazza dei Ciompi
Open: Monday-Saturday, 9:00-19:00

Description: Everything from grandmother's attic is found in this small flea market located next to Vasari's sixteenth-century fish market portico. Known as the **Loggia dei Pesci,** the portico was moved here in the nineteenth century when the old market around Piazza della Repubblica was demolished to make way for the formal square lined by porticoes.

Accessibility: There are lowered sidewalk curb cuts on all corners surrounding the market. The market pavement is rough in places. Doorways to most shops are wide enough to enter and, except for slight threshold lips, are either on a level or have makeshift ramps. Shops have crowded interiors, but objects are also displayed outside their doors.

Mercato di Sant'Ambrogio
Piazza Lorenzo Ghiberti
Open: Monday-Saturday, 7:00-14:00

Description: A colorful market frequented by Florentines; you will find fewer tourists here. Much of the fruit, vegetables, and flowers sold outside are produced locally. Outside stalls selling inexpensive and used clothing flank the north side of the nineteenth-century cast-iron market building.

Accessibility: The market building is wheelchair accessible on the east and west sides by long ramps with rough stone pavements. There is an elevator to the basement level to public restrooms, including a cramped, accessible restroom (door swings out) suitable for small manual wheelchairs only and then it's a squeeze. Cost to use restroom is €0,60.

Museo del Bargello (entrance may require assistance)
Via del Proconsolo, 4
Tel: 055 238 8606
Open: 8:30-13:50 every day except the third Sunday and third Monday of every month
Admission: €6,50

Description: Walking through the rooms of this very special museum is like retracing your steps through the Florentine Renaissance, especially when so much of the sculpture has been removed from its original setting to the safer, climate-controlled galleries of the Bargello. Not to be missed are the famous competition panels by Ghiberti and Brunelleschi for the Baptistery doors or Donatello's heroic *St. George* from Orsanmichele. Also memorable are Michelangelo's wine-sodden *Bacchus* and Giambologna's exquisite life-size birds in bronze, exhibited on the upstairs loggia, made for the garden grotto of the Medici villa of Castello.

Accessibility: There is a low step at the museum entrance (7.5 centimeters [3 inches]). A ramp leads from the main entrance hall into the courtyard. The accessible entrance to the ground-floor rooms with the Michelangelo statues is either from the main entrance hall or, if this entrance is closed, from the courtyard. For this wheelchair-accessible entrance, located behind the stone staircase, go counterclockwise around the courtyard.

An **elevator** is located in a room off the far end of the courtyard. Ask museum personnel to operate (door and cabin width: 79 centimeters [31 inches]; cabin length: 149 centimeters [58 5/8 inches]). Otherwise steep staircases with handrails lead to the upper floors.

An **accessible restroom** is located on the top floor. A guard must be asked to unlock the door and to operate the small stair lift (width: 68 centimeters [26 ¾ inches]; length: 86 centimeters [33 7/8 inches]; capacity: 150 kilograms [330 pounds]). Description of restroom— WC height: 48 centimeters (about 19 inches); horizontal and vertical grab bars on right wall; transfer space on left.

A few small ramps lead to some rooms on the second and third floors. Some stone door thresholds have a slight lip. Scattered seating.

Comments: Since the museum is short of guards, the third floor (*secondo piano*) is sometimes closed. While this does not mean you cannot use the restroom, it does mean that you may not be able to see the armor, the collection of small bronzes, or the magnificent della Robbia painted terracotta altarpieces. If you are interested in seeing these, call ahead of time to see if the third floor is open.

Museo di Antropologia e Etnologia (entrance may require assistance)
Via del Proconsolo, 12
Tel: 055 239 6449
Home Page: *www.unif.it/msn*
E-mail: *musant@unifi.it*
Open: Monday-Wednesday, Friday, and Saturday, 9:00-13:00
Admission: €4,00; €2,00 (children, students, people who are disabled)

Description: The origins of this museum date to the seventeenth century when the Medici became avid collectors of artifacts from the New World. The objects collected by them include a magnificent red feather priest's cap and the wooden sculpted bludgeons of the Tupinamba peoples from the Amazon exhibited in the last room together with mummified trophy heads whose mouths are sewn shut to prevent their souls from escaping. Even if you're not particularly interested in anthropology, this is a fascinating museum with life-size models of people and horses decked out in ethnic dress from Africa, Asia, and the New World, displayed according to nineteenth-century museum criteria.

Accessibility: The museum is located on the *piano nobile* (second floor). To use the elevator, ring the bell on the wooden gate to the left at the courtyard entrance. Museum personnel will come to operate the locked elevator which is located to the rear of the palace courtyard (door width: 90 centimeters [35 ½ inches]; cabin width: 138 centimeters [54 ¼ inches]; cabin length: 148 centimeters [58 ¼ inches]). Access to the museum is otherwise by means of a high, steep staircase located to the right of the main entrance door. There are no architectural barriers inside the museum. An **accessible restroom** is located on the ground floor in the courtyard on the left.

Comments: The elevator to return downstairs can be self-operated; its outside door is locked only on the ground floor.

Museo di Firenze com'era (conditioned accessibility at entrance; only with assistance)
Via dell'Oriuolo, 24
Tel: 055 261 6545
Open: Monday-Wednesday, Friday-Sunday, 9:00-14:00; closed on Thursday
Admission: €2,60

Description: While not on top of everyone's list, this is a nice little museum which describes the city's urban history. The model showing Florence during its Roman period, together with remnants of antique sculpture found under Piazza della Signoria, give a new dimension to understanding the Renaissance Florentines' fascination with their city's classical origins. Views of the city through old maps and prints and the collection of late sixteenth-century lunettes of Medici villas, meticulously painted by the Flemish artist Utens, round off the collection of Florence "as it was." Labels and explanations are in Italian, but a typewritten guide in English is available on loan at the front desk.

Accessibility: The entrance into the garden where the museum is located is highly conditioned by the sidewalk which has a bumpy stone surface with a downward slope towards the street and no curb cuts. There is a high lip (4 centimeters [1 ½ inches]) at the entrance gate threshold. The platform lift immediately to the left of the entrance gate does not work at present. Take the upward sloping gravel path leading through the garden to the porch where the entrance to the museum is located. Access to the porch is by an ill-fitting ramp; there is a second ramp at the museum entrance (base lip 2.5 centimeters [1 inch]). The museum is ramped throughout its ground-floor rooms. A decent, **accessible restroom** (grab bars; space for left transfer) is located off the big room to the left of the main entrance. The door to the restroom is kept locked. Ask a guard for the key.

Comments: Getting into and through the courtyard garden will require assistance. Once inside, this museum presents no architectural barriers. The restroom is clean with good accessibility.

Museo Horne (not accessible to wheelchairs)
Via dei Benci, 6
Tel: 055 244 661
Open: Monday-Saturday, 9:00-13:00
Admission: €5,00; over sixty-five €3,00

Description: The fifteenth-century Palazzo Horne, formerly Palazzo Corsi, lies in the heart of the textile district; in the basement there was once a dyer's workshop. Percy Horne, an English art historian and collector, acquired the palace towards the end of the nineteenth century and, when he died, bequeathed it, together with its contents, to the Italian state. In 1922, Palazzo Horne was reopened as a museum. Horne's impressive collection contains paintings, sculpture, pottery, glass, coins, furniture, and textiles including a predella painting by Masaccio, a triptych by the Sienese artist Pietro Lorenzetti, and a *St. Stephen* attributed to Giotto. VIVAT conducts tactile tours of the museum by appointment, also employing tactile maps to describe the neighborhood of Santa Croce and the architecture of the palace. (See "Museums, Music, Movies, and Sports" for further information on arranging tactile tours.)

Accessibility: The museum is spread out over the three main floors of the palace with no elevator and steep flights of stairs.

Santa Croce and Museo dell'Opera di Santa Croce (accessible with assistance)
Piazza Santa Croce
Tel: 055 246 6105
E-mail: *info@operadisantacroce.it*
Open: Monday-Saturday, 9:30-17:30; Sundays and holidays, 13:00-17:30
Admission: €4,00. People who are disabled and their companion enter free. Ticket includes admission to the church and to the museum.

Description of church: The Church and Convent of the Holy Cross or Santa Croce was founded by the Franciscan Order in 1228. In 1294 Arnolfo di Cambio, architect of the Duomo and Palazzo Vecchio, was commissioned to design a new church which was then lavishly decorated with murals, tombs, monuments, and stained glass windows by leading artists of the fourteenth, fifteenth, and sixteenth centuries. Giotto painted two narrative fresco cycles illustrating the lives of St. John the Evangelist and St. John the Baptist and of Saint Francis of Assisi, founder of the order (in the chapels immediately to the right of the main altar). Donatello made a remarkable *Annunciation* (1435) in gilded limestone (near end of right nave). The marble tombs of the humanists Leonardo Bruni by Bernardo Rossellino (next to the *Annunciation*) and Carlo Marsuppini by Desiderio da Settingnano (directly across in the left nave) are masterpieces of Florentine fifteenth-century sculpture.

Santa Croce is also the Florentine Pantheon, and since the fourteenth century, by special order of the commune, monuments have been raised there to honor the great. Michelangelo's tomb (in the right nave just inside the main entrance) is a somewhat disconsolate attempt by Vasari to design a tomb worthy of the artist he defined as "more divine than earthly." Macchiavelli, Gioacchino Rossini, Galileo, and Lorenzo Ghiberti, sculptor of the Baptistery's magnificent *Gates of Paradise*, are also buried in the church.

Accessibility: Main entrance involves ten steps (no banister). Near the ticket office on the north facade there is a ramped entrance leading to a secondary **wheelchair-accessible entrance.** The ramp has an acceptable 8 percent (1:12) slope but might be narrow for some at the turns. There is a short ramp just inside this entrance down to the floor of the church.

The nave and transepts of the church are on one level. The main altar and transept chapels are reached by nine steps (no handrail), including the Bardi and Peruzzi Chapels decorated by Giotto which are still partially visible from the level of the transept. High steps (20 centimeters [8 inches]) lead to the sacristy (five plus two steps; no handrail), the bookstore (five plus one steps), and the leather school (five plus one plus two steps) all reached through the large door at the end of the right transept.

Description of museum: The best things to see in this museum are in the first room, the convent's former refectory. The *Last Supper* by Taddeo Gaddi (ca. 1333) with an allegorical vision of the Crucifixion and scenes from the lives of SS Mary Magdalen, Francis, Benedict, and Louis of Toulouse is the prototype for the long series of *Last Supper* paintings or *cenacoli,* which decorated Florentine convent dining rooms. Cimabue's great twelfth-century *Crucifixion* is the most famous victim of Florence's last flood in 1966 when parts of the city were covered with as much as nineteen feet of water. The monumental bronze *St. Louis of Toulouse* by Donatello (1423) was commissioned to decorate the niche over the front door of Orsanmichele, but political vicissitudes had the statue of this famous member of the Franciscan order moved to Santa Croce where, for several hundred years, it decorated the church facade. Several of the mural and sculpture fragments on display were removed during Vasari's sixteenth-century renovation project to build the tabernacle-style large altars still visible in the church nave.

Outside in the first cloister is another highlight of the museum complex: Brunelleschi's **Pazzi Chapel** (begun around 1429), built as chapter room for the convent and private burial chapel for the Pazzi. The glazed terracotta decorations under the porch roof and the roundels of the twelve apostles in the interior are by Luca della Robbia. Considered the culminating achievement of Brunelleschi's career, the chapel embodies the same principles of architecture he laid out in the earlier Old Sacristy of San Lorenzo: a module is used to determine proportions; structural elements are defined by dark stone and the walls, built to enclose the space, by white stucco.

Accessibility: To enter the museum, there are two steps at the exit threshold of the church, followed by a staircase (fourteen steps; handrail) down to the level of the first cloister. A **wheelchair-accessible entrance to the museum** is located at Piazza Santa Croce, 16, to the right of the church's main facade. The sidewalk in front of this entrance has no curb cuts and is 14 centimeters (5 ½ inches) above street level. Once inside the wheelchair-accessible entrance, you will be in the first cloister. Follow the covered portico to the museum entrance on the right. The first and second rooms of the museum (the Cimabue Hall and the Stained Glass Windows Hall) are wheelchair accessible by means of short ramps with skid-free surfaces. To enter the following room with the Cerchi Chapel, you exit from the Stained Glass Windows Hall to the cloister portico. From the portico, there are two steps at the entrance to the Cerchi Chapel (highest step: 11 centimeters [just under 4 ½ inches]). The wheelchair-accessible entrance is found by following the portico around to the right into the second cloister. Once in the second cloister, turn right and go to the end of the portico to the level entrance into the Cerchi Chapel. From the Cerchi Chapel, a narrow doorway (69 centimeters [27 ¼ inches]) and ramp lead to the final two rooms. These rooms can also be entered from the bookstore; the entrance to the bookstore is located in the passageway between the first and second cloisters.

The Pazzi Chapel, located in the first cloister, has two high steps at entrance (each 18 centimeters [7 ¼ inches]). There is no ramp, but the interior is partially visible from the porch.

There is **no accessible restroom.** Seating is found in the Cimabue Hall only.

Comments: The roundabout way that one presently follows to move from church to museum and from one museum room to the other, together with the inaccessibility of the Pazzi Chapel, will hopefully be resolved by a restructuring project planned for the near future. Be sure to pick up the information pamphlet in English, giving a map and brief history of the church, either at the ticket office or at the entrance to the cloisters.

Nearest accessible restroom is at the tourist information office in Borgo Santa Croce, 29/r.

Sant'Ambrogio (accessible with assistance)
Piazza Sant'Ambrogio at the foot of Via Pietrapiana

Description: This parish church is one of the three oldest in Florence. The present structure dates to the thirteenth century with later interventions. Although the masterpieces that once graced its altars by Masaccio, Filippino Lippi, and Botticelli have long ago been moved to the Uffizi, its stark and beautiful interior, so typically Florentine, remains highly suggestive. The **Cappella dei Miracoli** to the left of the main altar contains a fifteenth-century marble tabernacle by Mino da Fiesole made to hold a miraculous chalice. A fresco by Cosimo Rosselli (1486) depicts a crowd in the piazza outside the church gathered in adoration of the relic for having delivered the city from the plague. In addition to the tomb of Mino da Fiesole located at the foot of the tabernacle, several other important Renaissance artists are buried in Sant'Ambrogio including Verrocchio, the sculptor; Francesco Granacci, the painter; and il Cronaca, the architect of San Salvatore al Monte; as well as some members of the Del Tasso family who were famous specialists in wood sculpture.

Accessibility: There is a ramp to the left of front door with **one step at the entrance** (12 centimeters [4 ¾ inches]). The width of door into the church is 70 centimeters (27 ½ inches).

Synagogue and Jewish Museum
Via Farini, 6
Tel: 055 234 6654
Open: November-March (Sunday-Thursday, 10:00-15:00; Friday, 10:00-14:00); April-May (Sunday-Thursday, 10:00-17:00; Friday, 10:00-14:00); June-August (Sunday-Thursday, 10:00-18:00; Friday, 10:00-14:00); closed on Saturdays throughout the year.
Admission: €4,00; €3,00 for groups of fifteen or more; the companion of a person who is disabled is admitted free.

Description: The green copper domes of the Jewish synagogue are a distinctive ingredient of the Florentine skyline. Built between 1874 and 1882 of white-and-rose-colored stone, its style, a mixture of Moorish and Byzantine elements, is similar to the architecture of other late nineteenth-century synagogues in Prague, Budapest, and Toledo. The museum, located on the second floor, traces the history of the Jewish community in Florence, beginning with the Renaissance, and displays an interesting collection of important ceremonial objects.

Accessibility: The synagogue and museum are wheelchair accessible. After purchasing your ticket and placing metal objects, including mobile phones, in small lockers (with keys) next to the ticket counter (security is very tight here), wheelchair users will proceed to the main gate for entrance. There is a stone walkway with a bumpy surface inside the gate, followed by a loose gravel path, leading to the entrance of the synagogue by ramp on the side facade to the right of the main entrance. A large elevator within the synagogue takes you up to the museum. Restrooms are located in the garden to the left of the synagogue, including a **wheelchair-accessible restroom** (use a coin to turn the lock; WC has fixed grab bar on right wall with space for left transfer).

Across the River: The Oltrarno

The Oltrarno, the "other side" of the Arno, is one of the city's most colorful neighborhoods. Antique stores and elegant palaces line both sides of **Via Maggio**, which, together with Via Romana, form the main artery leading from the city's southern gate of Porta Romana across the **Santa Trinita Bridge** into the heart of Florence's *centro storico*. Furniture restorers and artisans' workshops are clustered in the neighborhoods around the churches of the **Carmine** and **Santo Spirito** and in the side streets between Via Maggio and **Palazzo Pitti**. At the daily open-air market held in **Piazza Santo Spirito**, some farmers still bring their produce in from the nearby countryside, selling seasonal flowers, vegetables, and fruit from makeshift stands set up at the north end of the square. **Via Guicciardini**, lined with small shops catering to tourists, is the main route between the Ponte Vecchio and Piazza Pitti, a square built on the side of a hill and dominated by the impressive palace that was once home to the Medici. Behind the palace, the magnificent **Boboli Gardens** stretch up the hill towards the Forte Belvedere and down as far as Porta Romana.

Mobility

Getting There

Five bridges connect the main part of the historic district with the Oltrarno. From east to west, they are Ponte alle Grazie, Ponte Vecchio, Ponte Santa Trinita, Ponte alla Carraia, and Ponte Vespucci. The bridges have slopes at each end and will require assistance for most manual wheelchair users. Ponte alle Grazie and Ponte Vespucci are less steep than the other bridges. Ponte alle Grazie is convenient if you are coming from the Santa Croce neighborhood. Use the west side of the bridge and proceed along Lungarno Torrigiani to the Ponte Vecchio. Ponte Vecchio is pedestrian and closed to traffic. Try to avoid Ponte Santa Trinita which has high sidewalks with curb cuts that are difficult to negotiate and no curb cut on the west sidewalk off the bridge on the Oltrarno side. Ponte alla Carraia is the steepest bridge but has curb cuts on both sidewalks on the north bank and on the east sidewalk on the Oltrarno (south) side. Ponte Vespucci has curb cuts on the north bank of the river, but not on the south (Oltrarno) side. It's best to take the east side of the bridge which has a 4-centimeter (1 $5/8$-inch) drop from the sidewalk at the crosswalk in the Oltrarno.

Accessible Bus D, equipped with ramp and place (with tie downs) for one wheelchair, serves the Oltrarno area and leaves from the Santa Maria Novella RR station. The bus stop is located near the "Arrivals" entrance to the station. The bus passes near the American Consulate before crossing the river at Ponte Vespucci, continuing down Borgo San Frediano, along the riverbank to Borgo San Jacopo and past the Ponte Vecchio to Piazza Ferrucci. Return trip goes back to the Ponte Vecchio, turning into Via Guicciardini and making stops for the Palazzo Pitti, Piazza Santo Spirito, and Piazza del Carmine before crossing once again over Ponte Vespucci to the RR station. The bus runs approximately every eight to ten minutes from 8:00 to 20:00.

Buses 11 (wheelchair-accessible), 36, and 37 from Porta Romana cross the river at Ponte Santa Trinita. Bus 11 turns right at the end of Via Tornabuoni, heading towards the Duomo and Piazza San Marco. Buses 36 and 37 turn left at the end of Via Tornabuoni toward the RR station. Return trip from the RR station is across Ponte alla Carraia down Via de' Serragli to Porta Romana.

Getting Around

Piazza Santo Spirito is a pedestrian area, and Borgo San Jacopo has only limited traffic, but most of the rest of the Oltrarno has normal traffic flow. Via Santo Spirito, one block in from the river between Ponte alla Carraia and Ponte Santa Trinita, has been recently repaved and generally has little thru traffic. The sidewalks in Via Guicciardini and Via Maggio have been rebuilt with curb cuts. Most other streets in this neighborhood have very narrow sidewalks, and their uneven stone pavement makes for generally rough going, forcing wheelchairs sometimes to take to the street.

Taxi stands are located near the Ponte Vecchio in Piazza Santa Maria Sopr'Arno and just outside Porta Romana.

Designated parking spaces for disability permit holders are located in the two parking lots at Porta Romana. One lot is located just outside the city gate to the right (one space); the other is just inside the gate to the left (two spaces). Other convenient designated parking spaces are near the Ponte Vecchio in Piazza Santa Maria Sopr'Arno along the river; in the small parking lot at the end of Via Guicciardini near the newspaper stand to the left of the Palazzo Pitti (one space); and in Piazza del Carmine in front of the big yellow *palazzo* on the west side of the square. There is a private parking garage located near the Ponte Vecchio: Garage Ponte Vecchio, Via de'Bardi 35/45r, Tel. No. 055 239 8600.

To drive in this area of town, which is part of the ZTL (Limited Traffic Zone), unless you park at Porta Romana or the Garage Ponte Vecchio, you will need special permission (see "Driving Around" in the chapter on "Transportation").

What the Neighborhood Has to Offer

Just off the Ponte Vecchio on the left, you'll find a bar/tabacchi in Via dei Bardi, 74/r selling cigarettes, postage stamps, and bus tickets. Further down the street are the Golden View Open Bar, a restaurant, pizzeria, and wine bar all rolled into one that also offers Internet service, and a bank, the Cassa di Risparmio, both with accessible restrooms. Just opposite the bridge at the crosswalk is **Caffè Maioli** (accessible restroom; no grab bars). In good weather, you'll find outside seating in Piazza della Passera at the **Trattoria Quattro Leoni**, a popular eating place catering to the antique store crowd from Via Maggio (outside seating; one high step at entrance. There is no accessible restroom, but if you go at lunchtime, you can use the **public restroom** in nearby Via dello Sprone). There are a number of informal places to eat outside in Piazza Santo Spirito. **Ristorante Ricchi** (open for lunch and dinner with a special fish menu in the evenings) and its bar next door (with summertime outside seating; one step), serving *panini* and pasta dishes, has an accessible restroom. Closer to the river near the Ponte Santa Trinita in Piazza Scarlatti is the elegant, contemporary-style new restaurant **Beccofino** with outside tables and inside seating (9-centimeter [3 ½-inch] step at entrance; doorbell; accessible restroom). **Il Santo Bevitore** in Via Santo Spirito near Ponte alla Carraia is a less expensive and more casual place set in a spacious, rustic, vaulted room (accessible restroom with a vertical grab bar). Near the Brancacci Chapel just beyond Piazza del Carmine is **O!o**, a new place with accessible restroom open every day except Monday, 10:00 to 1:30 a.m., serving breakfast, lunch, and dinner. If you wander as far as Porta Romana, there's a small daily market just outside the gate where a *trippaio* sells delicious, hot tripe sandwiches over the counter to local workers and students from the art school located in the former royal stables beyond the iron gate.

Accessibility Checklist

The following list contains information on various places which are accessible to wheelchairs.

Accommodation

- Convitto della Calza
- Istituto Gould

- Palazzo Belfiore
- Villa La Vedetta (outside the city walls near Piazzale Michelangelo)
- Youth Firenze 2000 (outside the city walls near Ponte della Vittoria)

Places to Eat

- Beccofino
  Outside seating. Step at entrance.
- Café at Palazzo Pitti
- Caffè Maioli
- Golden View Open Bar
- Il Santo Bevitore
- O!o
- Ristorante Ricchi
- Trattoria I Quattro Leoni
  Outside seating. High step at entrance. No accessible restroom.

Accessible Restrooms

- Beccofino
- Boboli Gardens
- Caffè Maioli
- Cassa di Risparmio, Agenzia 12 in Via de'Bardi
  WC (51 centimeters [20 inches] high) has fixed grab bar on left with transfer space on right.
- Golden View Open Bar and Restaurant
- Il Santo Bevitore
- O!o
- Palazzo Pitti
- Ristorante Ricchi
- Via dello Sprone
  This is a public restroom located on a side street between Via Guicciardini and Via Maggio. Open 10:00-18:00; 9:00-19:00 in summer. Cost: €0,60.

Banks

- Cassa di Risparmio, Agenzia 12
  Via dei Bardi, 50 (near the Ponte Vecchio)
  Tel: 055 261 001
  There are two doors to this bank. For the wheelchair-accessible entrance, go to the second door from the direction of Ponte Vecchio and ring the bell (chiamata). Inside there is a ramp to the right. Go left at the top of ramp to the seating area in order to take a number for waiting your turn. The door in the corner of the seating area leads to an accessible restroom.

- Banca Toscana, Agenzia 15
  Piazza Pitti, 27/r
  Tel: 055 282 647
  There is an emergency exit to the right of the main door which can be unlocked. Since there is no doorbell, you need to alert the guard who is usually stationed near the entrance.

- Cassa di Risparmio, Agenzia 30
  Viale Petrarca, 120b/c/d (just outside Porta Romana)
  Tel: 055 222 333
  There is a short ramp at the wheelchair-accessible entrance. Ring bell to enter.

Pharmacies

- Farmacia Santa Trinita
  Piazza Frescobaldi, 3 (near Ponte Santa Trinita)
  Tel: 055 210 021

- Farmacia Gandini
  Via Senese, 8/r (outside Porta Romana)
  Tel: 055 221 744

Oltrarno

Monuments

1. Museo Bardini
2. Church of Santa Felicità
3. Palazzo Pitti
4. Church of San Felice
5. Church of Santo Spirito
6. Cenacolo of Santo Spirito
7. Church of the Carmine and Brancacci Chapel

Places to Eat

1. Caffè Maioli
2. Golden View Open Bar
3. Beccofino
4. Il Santo Bevitore
5. O!o
6. Ristorante/Bar Ricchi
7. Trattoria Quattro Leoni

Accommodations

1. Convitto della Calza
2. Istituto Gould
3. Palazzo Belfiore

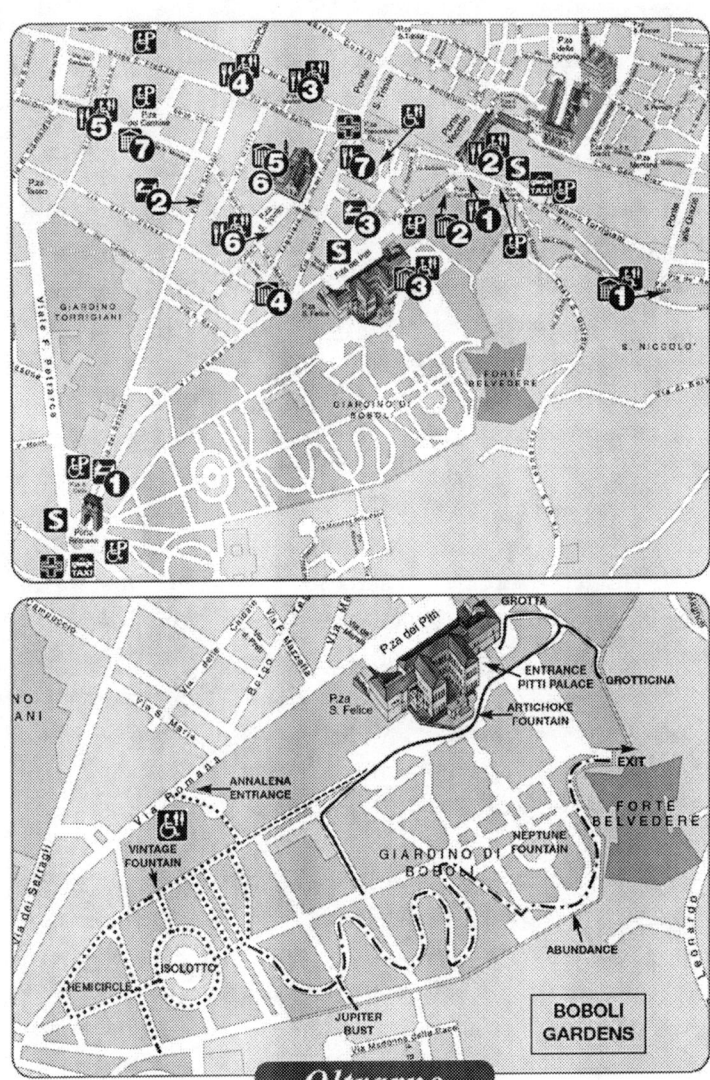

Oltrarno

What to See

Brancacci Chapel (presently not accessible to wheelchair users or to those who have difficulty climbing stairs)
Piazza del Carmine
Tel: 055 276 8224 for reservations and information.
Open: Monday, Wednesday-Saturday, 9:00-17:00; Sundays and holidays,13:00-17:00. **Reservation required.**
Admission: €4,00 with discounts for children, students, and people over sixty-five. Since only a limited number of visitors are allowed to enter the chapel at one time, there might be a waiting period if you arrive without making an advance reservation.

Description: Miraculously, the fire which destroyed the medieval Church of the Carmine in the eighteenth century hardly touched the recently restored Brancacci Chapel, one of the masterpieces of the Early Renaissance. The fresco cycle depicts scenes from the life of Saint Peter and was painted by Masolino and Masaccio between 1423 and 1428, completed some fifty years later by Filippino Lippi. Masolino's more elegant and decorative figures are still rooted in the International Gothic style, as evident in the *Temptation of Adam and Eve* and the scene of *St. Peter Curing a Cripple and Raising Tabitha* on the right. On the opposite wall, Masaccio's *Expulsion from the Garden of Paradise* and *Tribute Money* speak an entirely different language of naturalism, psychological realism, and correct use of one-point perspective.

Accessibility: Entrance to the Brancacci Chapel is through the door on the right of the steps to the church. An improvised stone ramp at the threshold may require some assistance. Reservations for visiting the chapel can be made at the information booth in the foyer. Proceed to the opposite side of the courtyard to purchase your tickets. The platform lift into the church located in the foyer opposite the information booth is not operating, and the chapel is presently reached by staircases only. The staircase to enter has fourteen steps with handrail, followed by two steps down to the

level of the church, then two steps up into the chapel. The staircase
to exit has eleven steps with handrail. The restroom (WC with
grab bars) is to your right as you enter the courtyard but has three
steps at the entrance.

Comments: If the platform lift was working, a wheelchair could
enter the church and, once inside, with the help of a few ramps,
gain access to the chapel. Unfortunately, repairing the lift only
solves one of the problems. The other has to do with the
apparent lack of cooperation between the city who administers
the chapel as a museum and the church. There is an interesting,
forty-minute film about Masaccio and his role in painting the
chapel (in Italian, French, and English) projected in the small
refectory off the courtyard, but this is small compensation for
not being able to see the real thing.

Cenacolo di Santo Spirito
Piazza Santo Spirito, 29
Tel: 055 287 043
Open: Tuesday-Saturday, 9:00-14:00 (summer); 10:30-13:30
(winter); closed on Monday
Admission: €2,20; sixty-five and over, €1,70

Description: The highlight of this small museum is the fourteenth-
century *Last Supper* by Andrea Orcagna, even though large parts of
it were lost when tall doors were cut into the wall to transform the
former convent refectory into a carriage house. The works on exhibit
belonged to Salvatore Romano, an antique dealer who bequeathed
this eclectic collection to the city of Florence. A Neapolitan, he collected
many pieces from his native Campagna such as the interesting animal
Romanesque sculptures of a lioness's head and the two sea lions
positioned under the fresco. Be sure to see the Tino di Camiaino
Angel and the two bas reliefs by Donatello from Padova.

Accessibility: The entrance to this museum is wheelchair accessible.
At present there is no accessible restroom; no seating.

Museo Bardini
Piazza de' Mozzi, 1
Tel: 055 234 2427
Open: Temporarily closed for renovation
Admission: To be established

Description: The antique dealer Stefano Bardini pieced together this neo-Renaissance palace in the nineteenth century (the windows on the *piano nobile* were originally altars from a church in Pistoia) to create a private museum in which to exhibit his collection. At his death, the palace and its contents, an eclectic collection of ceramics, carpets and tapestries, furniture, armor, pottery, sculpture, painting, and musical instruments was given to the city of Florence. Some of the highlights on display are the medieval statue of *Charity* by Tino di Camaino, the *Madonna dei Cordai* (Madonna of the Rope Makers) by Donatello, and Pollaiuolo's painting of the *Archangel Saint Michael.*

Accessibility: A new elevator will allow wheelchair access to the galleries on the main upper floor. Reopening is scheduled for sometime in 2004.

Palazzo Pitti (accessible with assistance)
Piazza Pitti, 1 (wheelchair-accessible Bus D stops directly in front of the palace)
Tel: 055 294 883 (Firenze Musei) for information and reservations
Open: For opening hours see individual museums below
Admission: Galleria Palatina (ticket includes admission to the royal apartments)—€8,50
Galleria d'Arte Moderna and Galleria del Costume—€5,00
Boboli Gardens, Museo delle Porcellane, Galleria degli Argenti—€6,00

Cumulative ticket valid for three days includes entrance to all museums—€10,50. The ticket office is located in the right wing of the palace flanking the *piazza.* Proceed directly to window 3 without waiting in line if you have reservations.

Description: Built for the banker Luca Pitti in the mid-fifteenth century, the Palazzo Pitti was acquired in 1549 by Eleonora of Toledo, wife of Duke Cosimo I de' Medici, who wished to move her children out of the gloomy, confining rooms of their official residence in Palazzo Vecchio. The palace stood on the edge of open land that stretched up the hill as far as the fortified walls surrounding the city. Its original nucleus, the seven central bays of the main facade, was gradually enlarged through the additions of a large courtyard and side wings, stretching out like two great arms out to embrace either side of the piazza in front of the palace. The land behind, once the site of a quarry which furnished the huge stone blocks for the palace facade, was developed into magnificent gardens, decorated with antique sculpture, grottoes, fountains, and an amphitheatre. Today six museums are located within the Palazzo Pitti complex which also includes the Boboli Gardens.

Accessibility: Manual wheelchair users will require assistance to manage the steep slope between the street level and the palace entrance. Follow one of the curving roads to the right or left of the *piazza*. The rough, bumpy stone pavement at the entrance and inside the courtyard, including under the courtyard porticoes, can be extremely hazardous, especially if you use a wheelchair.

The Galleria Palatina, Royal Apartments, and Galleria d'Arte Moderna are accessible to wheelchairs; the Museo degli Argenti has partial accessibility. The Galleria del Costume is accessible only to manual wheelchair users; the entrance to the Museo delle Porcellane involves stairs and is not accessible. The Carriage Museum, although accessible, is rarely open to the public.

An **accessible restroom** is located in the far-right corner of the courtyard next to the café, although it is antiquated, not heated, and may be difficult for larger wheelchairs to enter (WC has fixed grab bars to the right and rear, with transfer space on the left). Keys to this restroom are usually kept at the entrance ramp to the Boboli Gardens (to the immediate left of the restroom) and in the bookstore (directly across the courtyard). A second newer restroom is located upstairs in the Galleria d'Arte Moderna (fixed grab bars are located to the rear and right of the WC with transfer space on the left; unwrapped metal pipe under sink). Even if you do not wish to visit this gallery, ask permission from the museum personnel at the entrance to the gallery to use the restroom.

The **elevator** (door width : 90 centimeters [35 ½ inches]; cabin width: 139 centimeters [54 ¾ inches]; cabin length: 163 centimeters [64 ⅛ inches]) is located beyond the cloakroom off the right side of the courtyard.

One **manual wheelchair** kept at the ticket office is available for use of visitors.

Galleria Palatina (Palatine Gallery)
Tel: 055 238 8614
Open: Tuesday-Sunday, 8:15-18:50; closed on Monday

Entrance: On the second floor and reached by the grand staircase on the right side of the courtyard or by the elevator located beyond the cloakroom.

Description: The paintings in the gallery belonged to the Medici and date primarily to the High Renaissance and Baroque periods. Works by Raphael and Titian, Tintoretto, Rubens, and Andrea del Sarto, stacked one above the other against rich, damask-covered walls, still appear as they did at the beginning of the nineteenth century when the collection was first opened to the public. There are thirteen paintings by Raphael including the *Madonna del Granduca*, the Doni portraits and the *Madonna del Balducchino* all painted during the artist's Florentine sojourn between 1504 and 1508 when he was still in his twenties, while the *Madonna della Sedia* and the *Donna Velata* belong to his more mature Roman period. The five central rooms on the front of the palace and the *Sala della Stufa* overlooking the garden, ornately decorated in fresco and gilded stucco, were designed in the mid-seventeenth century by Pietro della Cortona, a leading Baroque artist who worked extensively in Rome. Explanations are in Italian only. Scattered seating is found throughout the gallery, and it is permitted to sit in the red velvet chairs.

Accessibility: No obstacles are found in the Palatine Gallery.

Royal Apartments: These sumptuously decorated rooms formed the private apartments of King Victor Emmanuel II during the brief period (1865-1871) that Florence served as the capital of the newly united Italy and continued to be used by the reigning Savoy family until 1912. You are allowed to stroll through, but not to sit. Be careful not to trip or catch a wheel on the runners laid down to protect the carpets. The apartments are located on the same floor as the Palatine Gallery, and the entrance fee to see them is included in the Palatine Gallery ticket.

Galleria d'Arte Moderna (Modern Art Gallery)
Tel: 055 238 8616
Open: Tuesday-Saturday, 8:30-13:50 and on the first, third, and fifth Sunday and second and fourth Monday of every month

Entrance: From the third floor of palace is reached either by the grand staircase or the elevator.

Description: This is an infrequently visited, but charming and very carefully curated museum for those who appreciate nineteenth-century Italian art. The collection ranges from neoclassical objects dating to the period of the French occupation of Italy, to portraits, history paintings, and landscapes including an important collection of works by the Tuscan Macchiaioli school. Some seating is available. Explanations and labels are in Italian only.

Accessibility: This museum presents no obstacles and has a very decent, clean, accessible restroom (WC 51 centimeters [20 inches] high; grab bars to right and rear; transfer space on left). Some of the smaller paintings exhibited in tall glass cases are not visible for small children or people in wheelchairs.

Galleria del Costume (Costume Gallery)
Tel: 055 238 8713
Open: Tuesday-Saturday, 8:15-13:50, and the first, third, and fifth Sunday and second and fourth Monday of each month

Entrance: Take the elevator to the third floor. As you exit from the elevator, turn right. The entrance to the gallery is down two short flights of stairs. See accessibility description below.

Description: Nineteenth-century court uniforms and neo-Gothic gowns worn by Florentine nobility for the costume ball held in 1887 to inaugurate the new Duomo facade are exhibited in charming period rooms overlooking the garden, followed by examples of twentieth-century costumes worn by famous people from the actress Eleonora Duse to Maria Callas. (On display until 2005. Main exhibits are changed every two years.)

Accessibility: Two short flights of stairs (total of seventeen steps) lead down to the entrance of this gallery. The gallery has a stair-climbing device which is suitable for manual wheelchairs only although a project to render the museum fully accessible is currently under study. Call the museum for further details.

Museo degli Argenti (Silver Museum)
Tel: 055 238 8709
Open: Every day except for the first and last Monday of the month; January, February, November, December, 8:15-16:30; March, 8:15-17:30; April, May, September, October, 8:15-18:30; June, July, August, 8:15-19:30

Entrance: Through the first door under the portico on the far-left side of the courtyard.

Description: The objects in this decorative arts museum once belonged to the Medici and reflect their eclectic and changing tastes in art. Highlights of the collection include Lorenzo the Magnificent's Byzantine and Roman semiprecious stone vases with their fifteenth-century enamel, silver, and gold mountings; the intricately carved and somewhat-bizzare seventeenth-century ivories appreciated by the later Medici; and the exquisite objects in *pietre dure*—vases, bowls, and plates—carved from lapus lazuli and rock crystal, many of which were once wedding presents or belonged to the dowries of Medici brides. The ground-floor rooms of this museum belonged to the palace summer apartments and are decorated with spectacular allegorical and *trompe l'oeil* frescoes. There is scattered seating in the front rooms where you will also find excellent printed explanations in English, French, German, and Italian.

The rooms on the mezzanine level contain collections of cameos, silverware, and some curious Mexican objects collected from the New World by Cosimo I de'Medici.

Accessibility: All ground-floor rooms are accessible, but there is no elevator to the mezzanine level. The mezzanine is reached by a staircase of four short flights of stairs (each containing between eight and eleven steps) divided by three landings and with a banister.

Comments: The most important objects are displayed in the splendidly frescoed rooms on the ground floor, making a visit to this museum well worthwhile even if you can't get to the mezzanine.

Museo delle Porcellane (Porcelain Museum)
Tel: 055 238 8605
Open: Every day except for the first and last Monday of the month (same opening hours as the Museo degli Argenti and Boboli Gardens)

Description: The pieces on display include examples of eighteenth— and nineteenth-century Italian, Austrian, French, and German china once belonging to the palace's post-Renaissance occupants.

Accessibility: At the highest point of the Boboli Gardens, the museum is located on top of a terrace reached by a long staircase (twenty-seven steps; partial handrail) and is not accessible to wheelchairs.

Boboli Gardens

Tel: For information in English on opening hours, call Firenze Musei: 055 294 883

Open: Every day at 8:15 except for first and last Monday of every month; summer closing time, 19:30; winter closing time, 16:30 with slight variations in the spring and fall (call to check for seasonal closing times)

Description: The gardens stretch up the hill behind the palace to the Belvedere Fortress and down to the right as far as Porta Romana. On axis with the palace is the seventeenth-century *Artichoke Fountain*, followed by an amphitheater where magnificent spectacles once were held to entertain the court, the *Neptune Pond* and, at the summit, a colossal statue of *Abundance*. In the garden's private reaches, rustic grottoes designed for Eleonora of Toledo and for Francesco I, her son, provided cool retreats during hot summer weather. The **Viottolone**, a long avenue lined with green cypress trees and antique white marble statues, reaches down the hill to a miniature island at its base known as the **Piazzale dell'Isolotto** with Giambologna's statue of *Ocean* in the center. Beyond lies a semicircular lawn decorated with two red granite columns. Amusing, rustic seventeenth-century statues of peasants, an abundance of capricorns (Cosimo I's zodiacal sign), and antique statuary are scattered throughout the garden. The garden is huge, and to see it all will require several hours. Benches are sporadically placed throughout but are especially concentrated around the **Piazzale dell'Isolotto**.

Entrance: There are four entrances to the garden: (1) at the Pitti Palace either through the palace courtyard or outside in the piazza through the gate in the left wing known as the Rondò del Bacco; (2) at the Annalena Gate in Via Romana; (3) at the Forte del Belvedere (only when exhibits are being held at the Fort. This entrance functions as an exit only); and (4) at Porta Romana (temporarily closed). The main entrance to the gardens is located in the far-right corner of the palace courtyard and involves a short flight of stairs followed by a steep ramp. The **wheelchair-accessible entrance** to the gardens is through the central door on the left side of the courtyard. If this entrance is closed, ask one of the guards on duty in the courtyard to unlock it or to indicate the Rondò del Bacco entrance.

Accessibility: Main garden paths have packed dirt surfaces covered with loose gravel. In most places the gravel is not deep, but in hot, dry weather especially, it tends to pack, making traction often very difficult. Wheelchair users will need an able-bodied companion to manage the paths; few of them are truly level since much of the gardens were built on the side of a hill. Wandering around the gardens without knowing where you are going can be a very frustrating experience because many of the paths have steps and steep gradients. In order to facilitate your visit, pay close attention to the suggested itineraries. Available maps indicate neither steps nor gradients, and signage along the paths is sporadic and gives no indication of accessibility.

Itineraries: The wheelchair-accessible parts of the garden can be divided into three itineraries. Depending on your stamina, on the time you want to spend there, and whether your chair is power or manual, you can follow a single itinerary, combine two itineraries, or do all three.

(1) The first itinerary includes the section of the garden to the left side and directly behind the palace. Entrance is either from the left side of the palace courtyard or through the gate in the **Rondò del Bacco** or left wing of the exterior facade of the palace facing the piazza. Important monuments in the first itinerary include Buontalenti's *Grotto*, the *Grotticina della Madama*, and the amphitheatre. Emerging from the palace courtyard, turn left and go straight towards the statue (copy) of Cosimo's favorite court dwarf *Morgante* astride a turtle which is next to the **Rondò del Bacco** entrance. The structure behind him is the terminal part of Vasari's raised corridor which once connected the Palazzo Vecchio with the Pitti Palace. To the right of the corridor you see Buontalenti's *Grotto,* constructed for Francesco I de'Medici (1583-1588). Due to a newly constructed staircase (eight steps) in the main path, the *Grotto* is now viewed from a distance by wheelchair users. A **handheld stair-climbing device** capable of carrying manual wheelchairs up to 150 kilograms (330 pounds) is available to reach the *Grotto* and is stored in the office next to the Rondò del Bacco entrance. The *Grotto's* unusual-looking facade is encrusted with shells, mosaics, and dripping stalactitelike formations, the Medici coat of arms and capricorns, the symbol of Cosimo I. Sixteenth-century statues of Apollo and Ceres are placed in niches flanking the entrance to the *Grotto* which consists of three rooms once painted wth frescoes and decorated with sculptures, fountains, sponge rock, and natural vegetation. Retrace your route to the path (6 percent gradient) leading up the hill between the marble-and-porphory Roman statues of the Dacian prisoners (second century AD). On the curve, go straight ahead through the formal small garden to visit Eleonora of Toledo's *Grotticina* (1553-1555). Return to the main path which winds past the rear of the palace and along the base of the amphitheater. From this point, you look in one direction straight up the hill, past the *Neptune Fountain* to the colossal statue of *Abundance.* In the other direction, the palace courtyard facade forms the backdrop to the theatrical *Artichoke Fountain* (1639-1641). From this point, the path slopes slightly upwards, continuing along the rear wing of the palace known as the **Palazzo della Meridiana.** The main path then descends towards the Annalena Gate and Porta Romana. Directly to the left of the main path and parallel to it, a secondary path leads you to a walkway vaulted with greenery and lined with benches. Go down this walkway to the edge of the **Viottolone** and, if the chain is down, into the *Viottolone* for a sweeping view down the hill to the lower gardens. Note: The **Viottolone** has a steep, downward, 16 percent-gradient slope. Retrace your path back towards the rear wing of the palace either to return to the palace exits or to take the main path down the hill to visit the lower part of the gardens or to exit at the Annalena Gate. This is a steep path with an 8 percent gradient and will require assistance. Continue straight down the hill to follow the second itinerary or turn right at the end of the iron fence and follow the descending path to exit at the Annalena Gate where you will find a wheelchair-accessible restroom (WC on pedestal base with transfer space on left; fixed grab bars on right and rear walls) located to the left just inside the gate and a ticket office on the right.

(2) **The second itinerary** includes the lower section of the garden from the Annalena Gate to Porta Romana. Important monuments include the **Piazzale dell'Isolotto**. Proceed from the Annalena Gate to the main path descending from the **Palazzo della Meridiana**. From the main path which now has a gentle slope downwards, there are several options for exploring the lower part of the gardens. The first, second, and third paths to the left lead to the bottom of the **Viottolone**. From here, turn right for the **Piazzale dell'Isolotto**. The fourth path to the left between the statues of two dogs and opposite the seventeenth-century **Fountain of the Vintage** leads directly to the **Piazzale**. All paths circling the **Piazzale dell'Isolotto** are level. From the **Piazzale** and on axis with the **Viottolone** proceed towards Porta Romana to the **Hemicycle**. The left side of the Hemicycle is obstructed by large tree roots and most paths to the left, as well as those leading towards Porta Romana, have upward slopes. At this point, in order to exit from the garden, you will have to retrace your route to the Annalena Gate or continue with the third itinerary.

(3) **The third itinerary** includes the top section of the gardens. Go to the bottom of the **Viottolone** where a carriage road to the right leads to the upper part of the gardens. The road (7 percent gradient) winds through uninteresting, wooded areas, but its meandering paths considerably reduce the steepness of the slope. Turn right at the first cross path and go to the end to view Giambologna's colossal bust of *Jupiter* (1560) and the bottom of the bizzare *Grotesque Masks Fountain* (early seventeenth century).

Return to the carriage road which will eventually bring you to the top of the gardens at the entrance to the **Viottolone**. Note: Heavy rains have washed out sections of the road, and while it is still transitable, in certain sections you must proceed with caution. Once you reach the summit of the hill, the indicated paths are all level or have relatively slight gradients. Proceed along the row of houses (on the right), bearing left where you see the steps to the Porcelain Museum and following the path in front of the *Abundance* statue. From this point, you have an excellent view down the garden's central axis towards the palace. Proceed in front of the statue bearing right towards the Belvedere Fortress (path is marked) to the exit. Note: Tickets to the gardens can be purchased three days in advance, and with advance purchase and ticket already in hand, one is permitted to enter the gardens at the Belvedere exit.

San Felice in Piazza (accessible for manual wheelchairs only and with assistance)
Piazza di San Felice (at the top of Via Maggio)

Description: San Felice is one of the oldest churches in the Oltrarno. A private gallery for the nuns of the convent next door was built above the entrance inside the main door. On the main altar is a recently restored early fourteenth-century *Crucifix* by a follower of Giotto. In the piazza outside the church, a column erected by Duke Cosimo I commemorates the victory at Marciana, a decisive battle in Florence's conquest of Siena in 1554.

Accessibility: There are two low steps to enter the church: one to the podium in front of church (8 centimeters [3 ¼ inches]); the other at the entrance threshold (6 centimeters [2 ½ inches]).

Santa Felicità (difficult accessibility and only with assistance)
Piazza Santa Felicità (at the foot of the Ponte Vecchio)

Description: Disembodied figures cluster in grief around a dead Christ in Pontormo's *Deposition*, a masterpiece of Mannerist art, which, together with the *Annunciation* and *Visitation,* appears in the chapel on the right just inside the front entrance. From the balcony built above the main door, the Medici could stop to attend mass as they passed, unobserved by their subjects in the streets below, along the raised corridor built for them in 1561 by Vasari to connect Palazzo Vecchio to Palazzo Pitti.

Accessibility: The wheelchair-accessible entrance through the doorway at Piazza Santa Felicità, 3, is very tricky, and you will need assistance. The ramp at this side door has a width of 83 centimeters (32 ½ inches) and a very steep gradient. Someone must first alert the custodian, sitting at the desk on the right just inside the church, to open the side door.

Santo Spirito (assistance advised)
Piazza Santo Spirito
Tel: 055 210 030
Open: 8:00-12:00; 16:00-18:00
Admission: Free

Description: Brunelleschi's project, approved in 1434, called for wrapping a ring of convex chapels around the entire perimeter of the church, including the main facade, thus bringing a new sculptural dimension to themes the architect had pronounced in his design of San Lorenzo some ten years earlier. Although the design was altered as construction continued after Brunelleschi's death in 1446, the interior of Santo Spirito remains one of the most harmonious in the city, and, with the exception of the large seventeenth-century *balducchino* over the high altar, time has not blighted much of its original decoration. The cool tones of the gray-and-white architecture frame large brightly painted altarpieces in each of the chapels. See the *Altarpiece of the Nerli family* (1488) by Filippino Lippi with its background view of the fourteenth-century city gate of San Frediano in the third chapel in the right transept. Of special interest are the original fifteenth-century *paliotti* or painted wooden altar fronts in the apse and transept chapels.

Accessibility: A ramp is located on the right side of church in Via del Presto di San Martino. Unfortunately, parked cars sometimes prevent easy access to this ramp. The wheelchair-accessible entrance is through the right door on the main facade by means of a short stone ramp with irregular pavement and an inner lip of 2.5 centimeters (1 inch). Once inside this entrance, there are two inner wooden doors: width 68 centimeters (26 ¾ inches). Use the left door for minimal maneuvering. The interior of the church is barrier free with the exception of two steps to the octagonal sacristy by Giuliano da Sangallo (1489-1492) and the magnificent vaulted vestibule (1492-1494) constructed after Giuliano da Sangallo's design by Il Cronaca.

Outside the City Walls

During Florence's long history, six different rings of city walls were built, beginning with the Roman settlement up to the fourteenth century when the last circuit was completed. Constructed between 1284 and 1333, the 8,500-meter-long fortified walls were designed by Arnolfo di Cambio with fifteen city gates and seventy-three defensive towers. For five hundred years, they stood intact until Florence became Italy's new capital and in 1865 were, in large part, demolished to make way for fashionable wide boulevards. Today anyone who wanders to the edges of the historic center can easily recognize where the walls once stood from the lone city gates and towers left standing in the middle of the busy multilane *viali*.

A number of things to do are located outside of the walls and lie within the range of a reasonable bus or taxi ride from the center of town. A classic stop on every itinerary is **Piazzale Michelangelo**, a panoramic vantage point built by the capital architect Giuseppe Poggi on the edge of a high hill upstream from the Ponte Vecchio. From the *piazzale,* you can see the city below locked in between two sets of hills on either side of the Arno. Beyond the boundaries of the *viali*, urban sprawl stretches east and west up and down the flat river valley while villas with olive groves and vineyards dot the green slopes of the hills to the north and south. The churches of **San Miniato** and **San Salvatore al Monte** are close to the *piazzale*. **Forte Belvedere**, an important part of the defensive wall system, still intact on the south side of the river, sits atop a neighboring hill. **Fiesole**, once an important Etruscan hill town, lies across the river to the north. The **Convent of San Salvi** with Andrea del

Sarto's splendid *Last Supper* in the convent refectory is located in a residential neighborhood to the east while to the west the **Cascine**, a public park, extends along the banks of the Arno.

To the South

Forte Belvedere (assistance advised for visiting the grounds)
Via San Leonardo at Porta San Giorgio
Tel: 055 200 1486 (for information on the exhibitions)
Open: Varies depending on the exhibitions
Admission: Varies depending on the exhibitions

How to Get There: If you have problems with mobility, taking a taxi is the best way to reach the Forte Belvedere which is located on top of a steep hill. Wheelchair-accessible Buses 12 from Porta Romana and 13 from Piazza Ferrucci stop near the other end of Via San Leonardo about half a mile away from the fortress but are not recommended for wheelchair users. The angle of the bus ramp is very steep since it cannot be positioned to rest on the sidewalk at either bus stop.

Description: Built around 1590 by the architect Bernardo Buontalenti, the Belvedere Fortress, as its name suggests, affords splendid views of Florence and the surrounding countryside. Forming an important part of the defensive system on the south side of the city, the fortress was also equipped with a special vault for the safekeeping of Medici treasures and, since it was connected to the Pitti Palace by an underground tunnel, served as a place of refuge in case of attack. Parts of the tunnel, in fact, were still used as places of hiding during the last world war. Today, during the summertime, Forte Belvedere hosts an outdoor movie theatre, and important art exhibitions are held there periodically throughout the year.

Accessibility: Forte Belvedere reopened in July 2003 after extensive restructuring which has rendered most of the exhibition space within the villa wheelchair accessible. An elevator is located to the left of the main entrance (door width: 80 centimeters [31 ½ inches]; cabin width: 110 centimeters [43 ¼ inches]; cabin depth: 135 centimeters [53 ⅛ inches]) which takes you to the level of the outside terraces and battlements. Exiting from the elevator follow the flagstone path to the side entrance of the villa.

The Villa: Just inside the wheelchair-accessible entrance is an **accessible restroom** (grab bars; right transfer) and an elevator which takes you to all three floors (door width: 80 centimeters [31 ½ inches]; cabin width: 135 centimeters [53 ⅛ inches]; cabin length: 138 centimeters [54 ⅜ inches]). Exit on level 0 for the bookstore and the two terraces. The paved terrace facing Florence has a ramp from the villa porch, and its low parapet permits views of the city and battlements below from a seated position. The grass-covered rear terrace is presently not accessible from the porch. On level 1, the galleries are arranged according to a circular route, but you will have to backtrack to avoid the high step at the exit in the last room. Level 2 presents no barriers. Two rooms at the main front entrance to the villa are inaccessible due to steep ramps and stairs.

The Grounds: A flagstone path leads from the first elevator, past the bar area and to the wheelchair-accessible side entrance to the villa. The path then continues beyond the entrance, going behind the villa and around to the opposite side, continuing in front of the villa to a lower level above the battlements. While portions of this sidewalk are new, others are older, and in some places the pavement is highly irregular. Negotiating the sections on the far side of the villa will require some assistance, especially since the pavement has a noticeable cross slope. Areas just off the sidewalks are covered with deep large-piece gravel. Most of the walkways along the edges of the battlements are inaccessible due to the presence of stairs or of highly irregular stone pavement.

Comments: The Forte Belvedere merits a visit for the spectacular view alone, and when there are important exhibitions, the bar/

restaurant setup on the grounds just outside the villa allows you the possibility of even having a light meal there. General policy allows free entrance to disabled visitors and to their companions. Although there is no designated parking space, those with permits are allowed to park inside the main gate near the ticket office. While the accessible restroom in the villa is generally well designed, the metal pipes under the sink are not wrapped, and the lock on the sliding door is very difficult to turn.

Piazzale Michelangelo
Viale dei Colli

How to Get There: Wheelchair-accessible Buses No. 12 from the direction of Porta Romana and No. 13 from the direction of Piazza Ferrucci stop at Piazzale Michelangelo. Both the stops for San Miniato and Piazzale Michelangelo on the No. 12 bus line are near sidewalks which permit a good perch for the bus ramp to rest on. The No. 13 bus from Piazza Ferrucci may present problems for wheelchair users since there is no sidewalk for the bus ramp to rest on which makes the angle of the ramp quite steep.

Description: Horse-drawn carriages have long been replaced by tourist buses, but the view remains terrific. Prices are steep at the *piazzale* even for an ice cream especially at the sidewalk cafés opposite the crosswalk. **La Loggia** restaurant (with wheelchair-accessible restroom) also has bar and café facilities where you can eat a sandwich. Accessible entrance is by ramp located on the left side of the porch as you face the building. There is an **accessible, public restroom** approximately 185 meters (600 feet) beyond the *piazzale* as you head in the direction of San Miniato. (Open June through September, 10:00-23:00; October through February, 11:00-17:00; March through May, 11:00-19:00. Small fee: €0,60.) A **taxi stand** is located in the *piazzale* near the crosswalk opposite the restaurant La Loggia.

San Miniato (accessible with assistance)
Via delle Porte Sante, 34
Tel: 055 2 342 731
Open: 8:00-12:30; 15:00-18:00
Admission: Free

How to Get There: Follow Via Monte alle Croci up the hill past the Church of San Salvatore al Monte, continuing in Via delle Porte Sante up to the fortified gate with the Medici coat of arms. Go through the gate. Immediately inside, there is an upward slope with irregular stone pavement up to the level of the piazza in front of the church. The church piazza has a relatively compact surface and is covered with small pieces of gravel.

Note: The road winds through a shady park provided with numerous benches. Total distance from Viale Michelangelo at the bottom of the hill to the entrance of the church is about 415 meters (1,360 feet).

Description: According to legend, San Miniato was an Early Christian martyr who managed to carry his decapitated head from his place of execution across the river near Piazza Beccaria to the hill where the Church of San Miniato was built. The present church was begun in 1018 and, like the Baptistery downtown, is an example of Romanesque architecture. Alberti turned to the classically inspired design of San Miniato for his design of the Renaissance facade of Santa Maria Novella.

The interior of San Miniato is impressive for its early thirteenth-century inlaid pavement with signs of the zodiac and for the inlaid pulpit and raised choir screen. The tabernacle at the end of the nave was commissioned in 1448 by the Medici and designed by Michelozzo, architect of their palace. Two of the capitals in the nave are spoils from local ancient Roman buildings. The Chapel of the Cardinal of Portugal on the left is an exquisite Renaissance "room" decorated by a team of some of the best artists working in Florence at the time. Vault ceramics are by

Luca della Robbia, the altarpiece (a copy of the original in the Uffizi) is by the Pollaiuolo brothers, as are the flanking angels drawing back the curtain; the *Annunciation* is by Baldovinetti. The sculptured tomb, of the young cardinal who died unexpectedly while on a visit to Florence in 1459, is by Bernardo and Antonio Rossellino. San Miniato is buried in the crypt while, above in the choir, a fourteenth-century panel painting tells the story of his martyrdom.

Accessibility: Entrance—Two ramps to the right lead from the level of the piazza to the raised stone platform in front of the church. The entrance door has two steps (16 centimeters [6 ½ inches] and 21 centimeters [8 ½ inches]). Hidden behind the right inner door you will find a heavy wooden ramp which can be fitted over the two outside steps. Note: The wooden support underneath the ramp fits over the first step. The inner left wooden door is wider: 70.5 centimeters (27 ¾ inches).

Interior: The nave has no architectural barriers, and it alone is worth the visit. Other parts of the church are reached only by staircases: nine steps (19 centimeters [7 ½ inches]) down to crypt; sixteen steps (18 centimeters [7 inches]) up to first level of raised choir; then one step (10 centimeters [4 inches] high) to area behind choir screen, and one step into sacristy (15 centimeters [6 inches]). **No accessible restroom.**

Comments: You will definitely need assistance with the ramp, both to put it in place and to maneuver it. The heavy wooden **ramp has a steep gradient and presently does not have a nonskid surface** which makes descent especially difficult.

San Salvatore al Monte (accessible with assistance)
Via San Salvatore al Monte, 9
Open: 7:00-18:30; closed 12:00-14:00 Sunday and sometimes on weekdays
Admission: Free

How to Get There: Take Bus No. 12 or 13 to the stop "San Miniato." The church is on your left as you follow Via Monte alle Croce up the hill towards San Miniato.

Description: Michelangelo nicknamed this Franciscan church *la bella villana* (the pretty country maid). While San Miniato is more spectacular, the austerity of San Salvatore al Monte, begun ca. 1490 by the architect Il Cronaca, is typically Florentine. His use of *pietra forte* or "hard stone" on the interior indicate the architect's desire to closely harmonize the design within and without. *Pietra forte*, in fact, was used primarily on the facades of Renaissance palaces such as the Palazzo Pitti, because as the name suggests, it is a durable, weather-resistant and, consequently, difficult-to-carve stone. The triangular pediments over the windows were inspired by examples of ancient Roman architecture that the artist had seen during his visits to Rome to study the ruins and were later used in window design by Michelangelo.

Accessibility: Entrance is through the side door which has one low step down (7 centimeters [2 ¾ inches]) to the level of the church floor. There are double wooden outside doors (each 57 centimeters [22 ½ inches] wide, with the possibility of opening both). Inside the side entrance are lightweight, double glass doors (each 60 centimeters [23 ⅝ inches] wide). Both doors can be opened.

To the North

Museo Stibbert (partially accessible)
Via Stibbert, 26
Tel: 055 486 049. Ticket office 055 475 520 for reservations and special requests
Open: Monday-Wednesday, 10:00-14:00; Friday-Sunday, 10:00-18:00; closed on Thursday
Admission: €5,00

How to Get There: The museum, located in a residential neighborhood about one mile north of the RR station in the direction of Via Bolognese, is best reached by taxi. No wheelchair-accessible buses serve this neighborhood. Bus 4 from the station stops in Via Vittorio Emanuele near the bottom of Via Stibbert, but it's a steep climb up the hill to the museum entrance.

Description: The Stibbert Museum, located in the former home of the eccentric Anglo-Italian collector Frederick Stibbert (1836-1906), is internationally known for its outstanding collection of costumes and armor. You'll find a bit of everything in the bizarre turn-of-the-century decorated rooms of Stibbert's villa which include over fifty thousand objects ranging from tapestries to ceramics, paintings and sculpture to the robes Napoleon wore when he was crowned king of Italy.

Accessibility: Recent renovations and the opening of a costume gallery have now made this museum 80 percent accessible. Entrance for wheelchair users is at the upper (north) gate, but an admission ticket must be purchased first at the main entrance in Via Stibbert, 26. An **accessible restroom** and **elevator** to the second floor are in the snack bar area near the accessible entrance.

Comments: Unfortunately, one of the best exhibits of the museum, the great hall with life-size warriors in armor mounted on horses, is not accessible to wheelchairs.

Fiesole

How to Get There: Wheelchair-accessible Bus No. 7 leaves from the RR station (the bus stop is opposite the "Arrivals" entrance) passing by Piazza San Marco on the way to Fiesole.

Description: Fiesole sits above Florence on a high hill offering spectacular views of the city. Founded by the Etruscans perhaps as early as the sixth century BC, it was one of fifteen major cities of the Etruscan League and occupied a strategic position of control over the mountain routes to the north. Later Fiesole was conquered by the Romans who built a small settlement there in the first century BC as testified by the remains of the temples, baths, and theater located in the park below the **Archaeological Museum**. During medieval times, the town remained independent until conquered by Florence in 1125. From the fourteenth century, Florentines began to build villas there, places to escape from the summer heat of the city in the river valley below: the setting for Boccaccio's *Decameron* was in a villa near Fiesole. On the steep slopes just under the town, Michelozzo built a villa for the Medici renowned for its splendid terraced gardens and magnificent view of the city below. Today Fiesole numbers around fourteen thousand residents and is a popular summertime destination hosting the performing arts festival *Estate Fiesolana*, held annually from June to September in the outdoor Roman theater.

Accessibility: Fiesole is built on the side of a hill, and few parts of the town are level except for the bottom of the main square known as Piazza Mino da Fiesole. For detailed information on the town's accessibility, see under "Fiesole" in the chapter on "Resources."

Museo Archeologico (assistance advised at entrance)
Via Portigiani, 2
Tel: 055 59 477
Open: Monday, Wednesday-Sunday, 9:30-17:00 (summer months until 19:00); closed on Tuesday
Admission: €6,20 (free admission for companion of persons who are disabled)

Description: This is an uncrowded small museum off the beaten path containing artifacts from Fiesole's Etruscan and Roman periods including some splendid bas relief fragments of Dionysian scenes found during the excavation of the Roman theater in 1873. The Costantini Collection on the second floor contains some interesting examples of Greek attic pottery, Etruscan bucchero ware, and some delightful provincial pieces from Magna Grecia such as the fourth century AD fish plate from the Campagna region in Southern Italy painted with depictions of fish, shells, and squid.

Accessibility: A loose gravel path leads from the main entrance and ticket office through the museum garden to the platform lift at the wheelchair-accessible entrance to the museum. Maneuvering the path at the main entrance may require assistance. All galleries are accessible by elevators or platform lifts (all minimum widths are 80 centimeters [31 ½ inches] with the exception of the lift to the Costantini Collection of vases—width is 72 centimeters [28 ¼ inches]). There are **two accessible restrooms**: one, on the top floor next to the bookstore; the other, at the main entrance opposite the ticket office. To exit from the museum, it is best to retrace your path to the entrance since the normal exit, by steep short ramp onto a narrow sidewalk on a hill, can be dangerous. The wheelchair-accessible entrance to the archaeological park is located near the parking lot in Via G. Dupré. Make arrangements with the museum personnel to open the gate. Much of the site is on hilly terrain with unpaved paths; only a few have gravel. Not recommended for manual wheelchairs.

Comments: Concerts and theatrical events for the summer festival *Estate Fiesolana* are held in the Roman theatre. Accessible viewing is from a terrace in the museum garden overlooking the theatre. For information call 055 597 8308.

To the East

Cenacolo di San Salvi (accessible with assistance)
Via di San Salvi, 16 (near the soccer stadium)
Tel: 055 238 8603
Open: 8:15-13:50, Tuesday-Sunday; closed on Monday
Admission: Free

How to Get There: Wheelchair-accessible Bus No. 20 (direction "Gignoro") from Piazza San Marco serves this neighborhood. Nonwheelchair-accessible Bus 6 (direction "Rondinella") passes through the center of town: Santa Trinita, Duomo, Piazza San Marco, Museo Archeologico with a stop in Via Lungo L'Affrico near San Salvi.

Description: This is one of those quiet, out-of-the-way museums that is well worth a visit to view an important collection of paintings by the High Renaissance artist Andrea del Sarto, including one of his masterpieces, the *Last Supper* (1526-1527) in the convent refectory. Admired in his lifetime as an exceptionally fine colorist and influenced by Ghirlandaio and Michelangelo, Del Sarto's harmonies of violets and pale blues, vivid reds, oranges and yellows are skillfully balanced in the *Last Supper* to bring unity to the different parts of the painting and to achieve a sense of quiet drama through use of color. Informative panels in both Italian and English provide descriptions of the major works.

Accessibility: If the gate is closed, ring *cenacolo* to open (high doorbell, 162 centimeters [63 ¾ inches]). A short path with loose gravel leads to the entrance porch with slight lip at entrance door threshold. There is a **stair lift** (68 centimeters [26 ¾ inches] wide; 81 centimeters [32 inches] long; weight capacity not indicated) which the custodian will operate for the small staircase (seven steps) just inside the entrance door. To view the *Last Supper,* enter the **Sala del Lavabo: one step at threshold** (4.5 centimeters [1 ¾ inches] up, then 11 centimeters [4 ¼ inches] down to floor level). The room which holds sculpture fragments of a Renaissance tomb by Benedetto da Rovezzano has **one step** down (14 centimeters [5 ½ inches]). An **accessible restroom** is located to the right of the entrance foyer. Seating is available in front of the fresco.

Comments: Designated parking spaces are found in Via Luciano Manara, 4 (first street to the right after you pass the entrance to the *Cenacolo*) and in Piazza di San Salvi in front of the *ambulatorio* (first-aid station). The bar at the corner of Via di San Salvi and Piazza San Salvi serves sandwiches and pasta plates at lunch and has an accessible restroom.

To the West

Parco delle Cascine
Piazza Vittorio Veneto
Open: Always; Tuesday, 8:00-13:00 for the market

How to Get There: Wheelchair-accessible Buses Nos. 12 and 13 run clockwise and counterclockwise, connecting the RR station to Piazzale Michelangelo, stopping near Ponte della Vittoria at the park entrance. Nonwheelchair-accessible electric Bus C runs back and forth parallel to the river between Piazza Vittorio Veneto opposite the park entrance and Piazza Piave near Ponte San Niccolò.

Description: The Cascine is a large public park running for three kilometers or about one and a half miles along the banks of the Arno in west Florence. The land now occupied by the park was once dotted with farms and a hunting reserve belonging to the Medici. In the eighteenth century, the Lorraine grand duke Pietro Leopoldo turned the entire property over to the public for a park. Today Florentines go there to jog and bicycle, walk their dogs, and stroll along the banks of the Arno. The park also holds a racetrack, the University of Florence School of Agriculture, a public swimming pool, and an exclusive, private tennis club. On Tuesday mornings, an outdoor market is set up along the banks of the river with over three hundred stands selling everything from cheese and salami to plants, porcelain, household goods, shoes, and discounted name brand clothing.

Accessibility: The entire park is on level ground, and a wide asphalt pedestrian street runs along the river. There is an accessible restroom in the park in Piazzale Kennedy, at the far end of the market near the foot bridge across the Arno (open June-September, 9:00-19:00; October-May, 10:00-17:00. Small fee: €0,60).

Medici Villas

The villa was a farm and place of recreation, a retreat to escape to during hot summer months and when dangerous plagues suddenly struck the city. The fifteenth-century Medici built villas to the north in their native Mugello, on the slopes of Fiesole above Florence, to the west at Poggio a Caiano and nearer the city at Careggi. Their sixteenth-century successors outdid them as testified by Utens's seventeen lunette paintings of Medici villas in the **Museo di Firenze com'era**. It seemed as though the ducal court was always on the move travelling from villa to villa, according to the changing seasons as they pursued their favorite pastimes of hunting and fishing.

How to Get There

The Medici villas of Careggi, Castello, and La Petraia are located fairly close to each other and are about a twenty-minute drive to the northwest from the center of Florence.

For the **villa at Careggi,** follow the signs towards Careggi, the city hospital. At the traffic circle called Largo P. Palagi in front of the CTO Hospital, follow Viale Pieraccini for about half a kilometer. The villa will be on your left and is not well marked. Enter through the great stone gate and park at the top of the driveway in front of the villa.

For the **villas of la Petraia and Castello and for Villa Corsini,** at the traffic circle called Largo A. Brambilla in front of the main entrance to the hospital, take Via Morgagni; follow the signs for Sesto Fiorentino and Castello turning right at the stoplight. You will be in Via Giuliani. After a little more than a kilometer, the road forks; take the right-hand fork (still Via Giuliani) towards Castello. Look out for brown-colored signs to Villa Petraia and follow them to the villa. The road is well marked. From "La Petraia," it is easy to find your way to the Villa Corsini and Villa di Castello. Take Via della Petraia back down the hill; the Villa Corsini is located at the foot of the hill in the small piazza. Opposite the Villa Corsini, Via di Castello leads to the villa which is about half a kilometer down this road.

The **villa of Poggio a Caiano** is located at Poggio a Caiano, a small town some seventeen kilometers from the center of Florence. Follow signs towards the A1 Autostrada and the airport at Peretola. At the airport, bear left as though you were heading back towards Florence. Turn right following the indications for Ponte all'Indiano, a bridge across the Arno. Take the first exit to the right for Via Pistoiese *before you cross the bridge*. At the stoplight, turn left into Via Pistoiese which runs straight through Poggio a Caiano. The villa is located on the right at the top of the hill just as you are about to head out of town. There is one designated parking space for disability permit holders in the small piazza across from the main entrance gate.

Where to Eat

Trattoria Zibbibo
Via di Terzollina, 3/r
Tel: 055 433 383
Open: Monday-Saturday, lunch 13:00-15:00, and dinner 20:00-23:00; closed on Sundays and in August

The *trattoria* is just up the street from the Villa of Careggi. Park in the small circular piazza at the top of the hill where there is one designated parking place. Entrance to the *trattoria* is on the left just a few meters down Via di Terzollina. **Two wide steps at entrance. Accessible restroom.**

What to See

Villa di Careggi (accessible with assistance)
Viale Pieraccini, 17
Tel: 055 427 9461
Open: Monday-Friday, 9:00-17:00; Saturday, 9:00-12:00; closed
on Sunday
Admission: Free

Description: The villa at Careggi was Cosimo il Vecchio's favorite
country home. There he enjoyed the simple pleasures of rural living
and could often be found pruning the grapevines and tending the
olives, planting trees, and conversing with the farmers. At Careggi
Cosimo also pursued his intellectual interests, spending hours in
his library or discussing Plato with the philosopher Marsilio Ficino
who owned a villa nearby. The covered parapet walk on the top of
the villa recalls medieval fortifications and was a motif used by
Michelozzo, architect of the Medici palace in town, in the design
of several other Medici villas in the Mugello. The irregular curving
facade is a reminder of the presence of an earlier structure,
incorporated by the architect into the villa proper. Today Careggi
houses administrative offices of the hospital.

Accessibility: There is a small lip at the iron gate entrance just
inside the main door. Turn left and enter the courtyard by means
of a small ramp. A ramp leads into the ground-floor rooms off the
courtyard. Upstairs rooms and loggia and the downstairs basement
room with the grotto are reached by staircase only and involve
many steps. There is **no accessible restroom**.

Comments: Restoration work is currently being carried out on the
villa, and at the time of publication, the gardens were closed. Unless
you are a particular fan of Renaissance architecture or of Medici
history or simply like poking around an old, run-down villa, a visit
to Careggi may be a disappointment especially since you can only
see the facade, the courtyard, and two ground-floor rooms with

fresco decoration dating to a period later than Cosimo. The best thing to see, the second-floor, decorated, open loggia overlooking the gardens is visible only on Saturday mornings and is off limits to wheelchair users.

Villa di Petraia (accessible with assistance)
Via della Petraia, 40
Tel: 055 452 691
Open: Every day from 8:15 to an hour before sunset (19:00 in the summer); closed the second and third Monday of each month; visits to the interior of the villa are conducted every forty-five minutes, beginning at 9:15
Admission: € 2,00. Ticket includes admission to the Villa di Castello. Free admittance for people who are disabled.

Description: Villa Petraia was built as a fortified castle in the fourteenth century by the Strozzi, longtime political and banking rivals of the Medici. Around 1544 it was bought by Cosimo I who in 1568 gave it to his son, Ferdinando. The architect Bernardo Buontalenti then transformed the former castle into a villa complete with the elaborate, three-tiered gardens seen today. In the early seventeenth century, Volterrano frescoed the central courtyard with scenes celebrating important events in the history of the family. Following a clockwise direction, you see the meeting of Medici Pope Leo X with the French king, Francis I; Cosimo I's triumphal entrance into Siena; Catherine de'Medici, queen of France; Tuscany's predominance over the Mediterranean under Ferdinando I; Lorenzo and Giuliano de'Medici received in Rome; Alessandro de'Medici crowned duke of Florence (the man in green is a portrait of the artist); Cosimo II receiving prisoners from the war in Bona; Maria de'Medici, queen of France; Francesco I de'Medici receiving homage in the Palazzo Vecchio; Pope Clement VII de'Medici crowning Charles I emperor.

Second noteworthy event in the life of the villa was its transformation in the nineteenth century into a hunting lodge for King Victor Emmanuel II during the brief time that Florence served as capital to the newly united country of Italy. For the occasion of the wedding of the king's son in 1872, the courtyard was transformed into a ballroom and covered with a glass and cast-iron structure. The furnishings of most of the villa rooms date to this later period.

Displayed in one of the ground-floor rooms is the Florentine sculptor Ammannati's *Hercules Fighting Antaeus,* a sixteenth-century bronze which once decorated a garden fountain at the nearby Villa of Castello. Outside in the garden on the upper level is the marble fountain of satyr figures by Tribolo leering at Giambologna's bronze *Naked Venus Wringing Her Hair,* brought to Petraia from Castello in the eighteenth century and now replaced by a copy for preservation purposes.

Accessibility: Villa La Petraia is perched on the top of a steep hill, and the main access to the villa, through the multitiered gardens, involves steep gradients, steps, and loose gravel paths. For the wheelchair-accessible entrance and for anyone with impaired mobility, stop at the ticket office just inside the main entrance and ask one of the guards to accompany you to a secondary entrance which will allow you to drive up to the rear of the villa. Entrance at the rear of the villa involves one step (19 centimeters [7 ½ inches]) into the courtyard. There is one step into the ground-floor rooms on the left of courtyard. The entrance into the room with Ammannati's sculpture is level. Access to upstairs rooms is by two flights of stairs.

The accessible upper tier of the gardens has loose gravel paths. From the terrace in front of the villa, there is a sweeping view of Florence and the gardens below. The park behind the villa consists of loose gravel paths descending and climbing through wooded and open areas.

Restrooms, including an accessible restroom, are located down a long flight of stairs. The **accessible restroom can be reached, with some difficulty, from a lower side entrance** to the basement of the villa, but since the gradient there is very steep, you must park the car next to this entrance and, accompanied by a villa guard, enter the side door and traverse long corridors with irregular stone pavements to reach the restrooms. An accessible restroom is also located at the nearby Villa of Castello (one step).

Note: The short route to the ticket office from the main gate is not accessible to wheelchairs, and either an able-bodied person or a call from a mobile phone will have to alert the guard to accompany you to the accessible entrance. As in most cases where a step is involved, the guards will willingly give assistance.

Comments: The best things to see—the courtyard fresco decorations, the Ammannati statue, and the Tribolo fountain— are on the ground-floor level of the villa and top tier of the garden. The lower tiers of the garden are actually best seen from above for once "inside" them you lose all sense of their geometry. The park behind the villa, while very beautiful, contains nothing of particular importance to see.

A complete new guide to the Medici villas, available in English, is for sale at the ticket office here or at the Villa di Castello.

Villa Corsini at Castello (accessible with assistance)
Via della Petraia
Tel: 055 23 575 (Soprintendenza Archeologia)
Open: May 1-October 1 (Wednesday, 13:30-19:00; Saturday, 8:30-19:30; Sunday, 8:30-14:00); November 1-April 30 (Wednesday, 8:30-17:00; Saturday, 8:30-17:00; Sunday, 8:30-14:00)
Admission: Free

Description: Purchased in the seventeenth century by the Corsini, important members of the Florentine aristocracy, this Renaissance villa was transformed by the Medici court architect Foggini into an exemplary model of late Baroque architecture. The facade, courtyard, and frescoed *salone* on the ground floor have been newly restored to hold part of the overflow from Florence's downtown Archaeological Museum. The extraordinary *Sleeping Ariadne* from Ferdinado I de'Medici's important collection of antique sculpture, once housed in the Villa Medici in Rome, has found a meaningful home down the hill from its collector's Florentine villa. The marble lion, a Greek original from the fifth century BC, was a popular subject of artist's sketches in sixteenth-century Rome. Important examples of Etruscan funerary art are displayed in the courtyard.

Accessibility: The entrance to the courtyard is level, and upon request, a wooden ramp can be put in place for the one step (19 centimeters [7 ½ inches]) into the ground-floor *salone*. Restrooms are upstairs, making the nearest accessible restroom at the Villa di Castello.

Comments: While not a Medici villa, the Villa Corsini is still connected to the Medici family by its contents and offers the chance to see some important sculpture in a beautiful setting. A division of the Archaeological Museum's restoration laboratory is housed upstairs and in some of the ground-floor rooms off the courtyard. Free parking is located in front of the villa.

Villa di Castello (accessible with assistance)
Via di Castello, 47
Tel: 055 454 791
Open: Every day from 8:15 to an hour before sunset (summer, 19:00); closed the second and third Monday of each month; visits to the interior of the villa are not permitted except by permission of the Accademia della Crusca
Admission: €2,00. Price includes admission to the Villa La Petraia. Free admittance to people who are disabled

Description: The villa at Castello played a central role in the life of Cosimo I de'Medici. It had belonged to his father and was the place he chose to retire to in his old age. When he became duke in 1537, Cosimo had Castello transformed into a residence worthy of his new role. The gardens were designed with grottoes, fountains, statues, and labyrinths, following allegorical themes signifying the glories of his rule. A great circular fountain was placed on the central axis of the garden. Decorated with Ammannati's bronze *Hercules Fighting Antaeus*, now at Villa La Petraia, the statue symbolized Cosimo wrestling power from his enemies to become duke. A shivering statue of *Apennine* in the upper wooded part of the garden, also by Ammannati, represents January, the month of Cosimo's election. The bizarre animal grotto decorated with sponges, shells, stalactites, and exotic animals—lions, giraffes, elephants, and a unicorn made of stone and polychrome marble—once included Giambologna's bronze birds, now displayed on the upper loggia of the Bargello Museum. Originally decorated with an image of Orpheus, the poet who could charm wild beasts with the sound of his lyre, the grotto alluded to Cosimo's abilities to pacify his enemies.

Accessibility: The lower formal gardens consist of upward-sloping, loose gravel paths. Surfaces of the larger side paths are more compact and lead directly to the top level with the animal grotto, otherwise reached by a short staircase on the central axis. To reach the upper wooded garden, take the three-flight staircase to the left of the grotto or return to the entrance of the formal garden and take one of the winding paths leading uphill to the left. An **accessible restroom** is located just inside the main entrance beyond the ticket office on the left: one high step at entrance (16.5 centimeters [6 ½ inches]).

Comments: Don't be disappointed if you are not able to get inside this villa even though Botticelli's *Primavera* and *Birth of Venus* once decorated its rooms. Those famous paintings are now in the Uffizi, and the garden, which set the prototype for other famous Renaissance gardens, is really the important thing to see.

Villa di Poggio a Caiano (accessible with assistance)
Piazza dei Medici, 14
Poggio a Caiano
Tel: 055 788 012
Open: Every day, except the second and third Monday of the month. January, February, November, December, 8:15-16:30; March, 8:15-17:30; April, May, September, and October, 8:15-18:30; June-August, 8:15-19:30; tickets are sold up until one hour before closing time; visits to see the villa interior are conducted every hour on the half hour from 8:30 to one hour before closing time (the schedule may be reduced during the winter months)
Admission: €2,00. Free admittance for people who are disabled.

Description: Lorenzo the Magnificent purchased the property at Poggio a Caiano in 1479, developing the land into a productive dairy farm and enlarging and transforming a preexisting medieval structure into a villa. Giuliano da Sangallo, his favorite architect, used a classical temple front motif for the porch on the main facade, and his design was famous enough to attract a probable visit by Palladio in the sixteenth century. Echoes of Poggio a Caiano's design from the temple front facade to its symmetrical plan are underlying themes in many Palladian villas.

The nineteenth-century, neoclassic interiors of many rooms date from the time when King Victor Emmanuel II lived at Poggio a Caiano, while the more interesting decorations belong to the Medici period. The walls of the barrel-vaulted huge central *salone* on the main floor are decorated with frescoes celebrating four generations of Medici rule whose lives are paralleled with figures from Roman history. See Andrea del Sarto's *Tribute to Augustus Caesar* where the seated emperor is being presented with gifts of animals, including an anachronous New World turkey. The Augustan Age known as the "Golden Age of Peace" was drawn as parallel to the Medici Pope Leo X's papacy. In Jacopo Pontormo's lunette painting of *Vertumnus and Pomona* (1519-1521) country peasants and a dog are perched on a ledge too shallow to hold them in deliberate contradiction of spatial illusion, typical of the artist's Mannerist style. Andrea Sansovino's ceramic frieze has been removed from the outside porch and is now displayed in one of the front side rooms. Complicated themes are woven into an allegory of time: eternity is represented by a snake eating its tail, while nature gives birth to souls. The two-headed Janus looks backwards and forwards as Mars emerges from a temple doorway to symbolize the Florentine New Year which began on the 25th of March.

Accessibility: One designated parking place is located in the small piazza across the street from the main entrance. An irregular, bumpy stonewalk outside the main gate leads left to the ticket office at the entrance to the grounds. Leaving the ticket office, there is one step (9 centimeters [3 ½ inches]) up to the level of the garden surrounding the villa. Slightly sloping gravel paths lead to the front and right side of the villa where a formal *giardino all'italiano* is found. Behind the villa, steep paths lead down to wooded areas. An **accessible restroom** is located on the main floor of the villa near the elevator (elevator door width just under 1 meter [approximately 39 ¼ inches]). On the second floor (*piano nobile*), two high steps lead down to the level of the front porch where reproductions of Sansovino's frieze have replaced the original ceramic panels. You might ask the guard if you can use one of the ramped emergency exit doors in the main *salone* in order to see the porch.

Comments: Of the three Medici villas, this is the easiest to visit for wheelchair users. The gardens are historically less interesting but do not involve lots of sloping paths, except in the rear, as they do at Villa di Castello, and because there is an elevator, you get to see more of the interior than you do at Villa la Petraia.

Museums, Music, Movies, and Sports

Museums

Making Reservations for State-Owned Museums:

Reservations can be made for the following museums. In order to avoid waiting in long lines, this is especially recommended for the Accademia, the Uffizi and, during high tourist season, the museums at the Pitti Palace:

- **Galleria dell'Accademia**
- **Galleria degli Uffizi**
  Galleria Palatina as well as all other museums in the Pitti Palace, including the **Boboli Gardens**
- **Museo Archeologico**
- **Museo di San Marco**
- **Cappelle Medicee** (not wheelchair accessible)
- **Museo del Bargello**
- **Museo dell'Opificio delle Pietre Dure**

For reservations, call Firenze Musei: 055 294 883. Monday-Friday, 8:30-18:00; Saturday, 8:30-13:00 (Italian time). Fax: 055 264 406; E-mail: *operapren@tin.it*.

The procedure is as follows: Upon calling, you will be given a reservation number for the reservations you make in each museum. Present yourself at the museum fifteen to thirty minutes before the time of your reservation. Do not wait in line but go directly to the reservation desk where you will pick up and pay in cash for your reserved tickets in addition to a small charge for the reservation. Cost per reservation per person is €3,00.

Guided tours for visitors with visual impairments: VIVAT (Volontari Italiani Visite Artistiche Tattili) offers, also for English-speaking visitors, tactile guided tours at the following museums: Cappella Rucellai, Museo Horne, Museo dell'Opera del Duomo, Museo Marino Marini, Museo di Paleontologia, and at the Museo del Tessuto in Prato. For further information and reservations which must be made at least twenty days prior to the visit, contact VIVAT, Museo Marino Marini, Piazza San Pancrazio, 50123 Florence, Tel. No. 055 219 432, Fax: 055 289 510 or E-mail: *vivatfirenze@virgilio.it.*

A limited number of wheelchairs are available for use in the following museums: Galleria dell'Accademia, Galleria degli Uffizi, the museums in the Pitti Palace, Palazzo Vecchio. For further explanation, see individual listings.

Museum hours are subject to frequent change. For the latest information, call the individual museums or a tourist information office.

Museum ticket offices close between an hour to one-half hour before closing time. Times are set at the discretion of each museum.

Some museums offer reductions for children, students, adults over sixty-five, and to people who are disabled and to their companions.

Music and Dance

Florence has a lively classical musical agenda each year. The major theater is the **Teatro Comunale**, officially known as the Teatro del Maggio Musicale Fiorentino, which holds a concert season from January through March, an opera and ballet season from October through December, and in the intervening spring and summer months, events from the annual "Maggio Musicale" Music Festival. **Teatro della Pergola**, one of Italy's oldest theaters founded in 1656, holds concerts organized by the Amici della Musica and small-scale opera performances for the Maggio Musicale Fiorentino. **Teatro Verdi** is the home of the Orchestra Regionale Toscana (ORT), a relatively new orchestra founded in 1980 whose program reflects Baroque through modern music with an emphasis on nineteenth-century works. Reservations can be made either directly at the respective theaters or through the Box Office ticket agency (see "Reservations" in the chapter on "General Information and Practical Tips").

Teatro Comunale
Corso Italia, 16
Tel: 055 213 535
Fax: 055 287 222
Home Page: *www.maggiofiorentino.com*

Accessibility: There is a short ramp in front of the furthest door to the right at the main entrance. One box (No. 3) with wider door (70 centimeters [27 ½ inches]) can accommodate up to four wheelchairs with seating for companions. There is an **accessible restroom** outside the main lobby near the entrance to the Piccolo Teatro. Restroom has horizontal grab bars to left of WC (52 centimeters [20 ½ inches] high) with retractable grab bar on right and room for right transfer. The Piccolo Teatro is accessible from the side entrance, and you will need to be accompanied there. The ground-floor bar area is accessible.

Teatro della Pergola
Via della Pergola, 12/32
Tel: 055 226 4316

E-mail: *teatro@pergola.firenze.it*
Home Page: *www.pergola.firenze.it*

Accessibility: Currently there are two options for attending events at the Teatro della Pergola while, in the near future, plans to build a new elevator will permit access to all levels of the theater from the parterre to the upper-tier galleries. At present it is possible to sit either in the parterre or in one of the first tier boxes. For access to the parterre, go to the wheelchair-accessible entrance in Via della Pergola, 18. The parterre is reached by a steep ramp with one step (17 centimeters [6 ¾ inches]) at the top of the ramp, assisted by trained *vigili del fuoco* (members of the Fire Department) and members of the theater staff. You may either transfer to a seat or remain in your wheelchair. A theater attendant is on duty throughout the performance should you need assistance. An **accessible restroom** is located nearby in the outside corridor opposite the ramp into the parterre. Ample-sized restroom has grab bars to the left and right rear of the WC (height approximately 51 centimeters [20 inches]), transfer space from right.

To sit in a first tier box, you must go to the entrance in Vicolo della Pergola, 2 (a small dead-end street to the left of the main entrance to the theater). You can drive into this street to unload passengers but cannot park here. A theater attendant will accompany you to the elevator. The elevator measures 138 by 138 centimeters (54 ³/₈ by 54 ³/₈ inches) and has two doors (78 centimeters [30 ¾ inches] wide) placed at right angles. Exit on the upper floor is to the right. The boxes are quite small and have room for two wheelchairs. The door to the box is 66 centimeters (26 inches) wide. There is a wheelchair-accessible restroom on this level: the WC (51 centimeters [20 inches] high) has horizontal grab bars along the right and back walls with transfer space from the left side.

When making reservations, be sure to specify if you are on a wheelchair in order to have proper seating and to alert the theater personnel to be on hand for assistance. People who are disabled and their companions are both entitled to a 40 percent discount.

Teatro Verdi
Via Ghibellina, 99
Tel: 055 212 320
Home Page: *www.teatroverdifirenze.it*

Accessibility: There is a short ramp at the main entrance in Via Ghibellina (furthest door to the right). Once inside the theater, ask one of the attendants to accompany you to the ramp leading to the upper section of the lobby. This ramp, which is behind a closed door, has a cross slope and may require assistance. In the upper part of the lobby near the top of the ramp is a **wheelchair-accessible restroom.** Space is sufficient in the restroom, but the close proximity of the support bars to either side of the WC (46 centimeters [18 inches] high) make transfer possible from the front only. Entrance to the parterre is by a steep long ramp and may require assistance. A ramped fire exit is located directly opposite this ramp. For the performance, you may either remain in your wheelchair or transfer to an aisle seat. The companion of the person who is disabled enters free. Future plans call for the construction of an accessible new restroom. Call the theater for further information.

Movies in English

Cinema Odeon
Via Sassetti, 1
Tel: 055 214 068
Home Page: *www.cinehall.it*

Description: Recent films are projected in their original language Monday, Tuesday, and Thursday.

Accessibility: The wheelchair-accessible entrance is in Piazza Strozzi, 7/r, but you must first alert the ticket office to open the door. There is a high sidewalk curb and one step at the main entrance and ticket office in Via Sassetti. **No accessible WC** (the nearest would be those of the Rinascente Department Store and Hotel Savoy in Piazza della Repubblica).

Cinema Fulgor
Via Maso Finiguerra, 24/r
Tel: 055 238 1881

Description: A recent film is projected every Thursday at this cinema located two blocks in from Ponte Vespucci.

Accessibility: All five theaters are wheelchair accessible, some with stair lift, but the film in English is usually shown in one of the ground-floor theaters. There is a **wheelchair-accessible WC.**

Sports

Stadio Comunale Artemio Franchi
Via M. Fanti
Tel: 055 503 121 (for information on free tickets to the games for people who use a wheelchair)
Home Page: *www.fiorentina.it* for schedules of games (in Italian)

Description: The city stadium and home of the local soccer team known as "La Fiorentina" or "La Viola" (color of the players' uniforms) is also an important modern-engineering feat in reinforced concrete designed in1931 by Pier Luigi Nervi. Attending a soccer game in Florence can be a real experience, especially when the arch rival team from Turin, Juventus, is in town. Tickets for the games can be purchased at the Chiosco degli Sportivi in Via Anselmi near Piazza della Repubblica and from the Box Office ticket agency (see chapter on "General Information and Practical Tips"). People in wheelchairs and their companions are entitled to free tickets.

Accessibility: Restructuring of the stadium in 1990 included building some wheelchair-accessible restrooms and covered viewing areas specifically designated for spectators in wheelchairs. There are about 125 places, and they're not always available, so try to call well ahead of time to see if you can get in. Enter from the west side through one of the gates for the Parterre di Tribuna.

General Information and Practical Tips for Visiting Florence

The following information, arranged in alphabetical listings, gives some general information and practical tips for visiting Florence. Understanding that you have to hail a bus but not a cab, how to locate a decent (and accessible) restroom, use a telephone, or figure out the complicated street-numbering system, should help to make your visit a lot easier.

Climate

Florence sits in a river valley between two sets of hills and tends to capture not only heat, but also cold and dampness. The city does not always have an ideal climate. Often extremely hot in July and August, rainy in November, or with a cold snap in December or January, it's best to visit Florence in the springtime (April, May, and early June) or in autumn (mid-September through October). The crowded and expensive tourist season runs from Easter through September while the city is comparatively less costly and empty of tourists in November, most of December, January, February, and early March. Due to the now-unpredictable global climate, in most seasons, it is advisable to dress in layers.

Communication

Internet points

Located throughout the city. The few listed below are accessible to wheelchair users but do not have accessible restrooms.

- **Internet Train** in the underground gallery at the station of Santa Maria Novella. Tel. No. 055 239 9729. Take the stair lift on the staircase at the "Arrivals" side of the station down to the gallery or the elevator, located inside the station opposite the ticket counters. The Internet point is located on the left in the main section of the gallery opposite the stairs. A ramped entrance to the gallery is located in Piazza Unità next to the Hotel Baglioni.
- **Internet Train** in Via de'Benci, 38/r, close to Piazza Santa Croce. Tel. No. 055 263 8555. Door at entrance: 80 centimeters (31 ½ inches) wide with 2.5-centimeter (1-inch) lip and encased doormat. Height of computer tables: 71 centimeters (28 inches). No accessible restroom, but the tourist information office with accessible restroom in Borgo Santa Croce, 29/r, is nearby.
- **Internet Train** in Borgo la Croce, 33/r, near the Sant'Ambrogio Market. Tel. No. 055 234 7852. Level entrance from sidewalk. Sidewalk curb: 12 centimeters (4 ¾ inches). There is a lowered curb cut on the sidewalk at the corner of Piazza Beccaria and Borgo la Croce but in some places the sidewalk narrows to around 72 centimeters (28 ³/₈ inches).
- **Internet Service** in Piazza della Signoria, 37/r. Tel. No. 055 214 914. Main entrance has one step down. The wheelchair-accessible entrance is around the corner in Via dei Magazzini, 1. You will have to ask them to unlock the door.

Post Offices and Mailing

Stamps can either be bought in any *tabaccheria* (tobacco shop) or post office. Priority mail (*posta prioritaria*) gets your letter out faster. Calculate around four or five days for a letter to arrive in the USA, three days in Europe, one day in Italy. Sending a letter or postcard weighing twenty grams or under costs €0,60 cents for Italy or Europe; €0,80 cents for the States. Postboxes are red and mainly located outside the city post offices. All mail to a destination other than Florence goes into the *altre destinazioni* (other destinations) slot and in the appropriate *posta prioritaria* box, if you have chosen this surer, faster service.

There are two main city post offices: one located in Via Pellicceria, 3 (just off Piazza della Repubblica), which is open Monday-Friday, 8:15-19:00, and on Saturday, 8:15-12:30. Wheelchair-accessible entrance is from the rear in Via de' Sassetti, 2. The other post office is in Via Pietrapiana, 53 (corner Via Verdi) which is open Monday-Friday, 8:15-19:00 and on Saturday, 8:15-12:30.

Telephone

- **Dialing**

To dial a number in Italy, you always include the local area code before the number; thus to call a taxi in Florence, dial 055 (area code), followed by the number 4390. Local numbers can be of four, five, six, or seven digits. Numbers beginning with 800 are toll free (*numero verde*). For operator assistance for both national and international calls, dial 170; for directory assistance, 12; for international directory assistance, 176; for wake-up calls, 4114. Emergency numbers to call for medical help, the ambulance, police or fire department require no area code and are the same throughout Italy. To dial Italy from abroad, you first dial the exit code (from the States, 011; from the UK, 00) followed by the country code for Italy (39), then the area code of the city you are calling, followed by the number. To call abroad from Italy, use the exit code 00.

- **Public Phones**

Locating a public telephone that works in a country with one of the highest number of mobile phones in Europe can sometimes be very frustrating. If you cannot find a phone which works on the street, look for a bar, restaurant, or tobacco shop with a red telephone insignia posted outside the door. Using a public phone can be another adventure. Instead of using coins, most phones now operate with telephone cards (*scheda telefonica*) which can be bought at bars, newspaper stands, and tobacco shops. Sometimes in a bar or restaurant, you will find a metered phone. You need to ask for the line and, after you finish talking, pay for the call.

- **Mobile Phones**

Mobile phones can be rented in the center of town from Platform 3000 in Via Ghibellina, 178/r (near the Bargello Museum). Open Monday-Friday, 10:00-19:00. Tel. No. 055 265 8117. Home page: www.platform3000.com. Click on "wireless phones." This company has an agreement with Piccell Wireless, an American company, and a phone also can be shipped to your home before you leave; you can travel with it all over Europe and ship it back once you reach home. If you plan to pick up a phone in Florence, however, the entrance to the office has three steps.

Currency

As of February 2002, the Italian lira was replaced by the European euro. There are bank notes for €5, €10, €20, €50, €100, €200, and €500 and coins for 1, 2, 5, 10, 20, 50 cents and €1 and €2. In expressing numerical amounts in euro, in Italy commas and periods are used in the following way. A comma is used to separate euro from cents, thus five euro and twenty-six cents is written as 5,26 while one thousand euro is written as 1.000,00. For current exchange rates see *www.xe.com/ict*.

Electric Current

Italy, like the rest of Europe, operates on 220-volt electricity. Small appliances like hair dryers often have a switch which coverts from US-standard 110-volt to the 220-volt electricity used in Europe. If your hair dryer does not have the converter switch, in order to operate it, you will need a small transformer. Concerning power wheelchairs, it is probably best to buy a universal wheelchair battery charger with settings for 110 and 220 volts. A decent, lightweight, inexpensive small charger with dual settings is available for about $160 from MK Battery (*www.mkbattery.com*). If you do not choose to purchase the charger, you will then need to have a reliable converter or transformer.

Italian plugs have two or three round prongs with all prongs in a straight line. It is easiest to buy a plug adapter at a travel store in the States before leaving. A plug adapter can be found in Florence at Cecchi Mario and Figli, Via Sant'Elizabetta, 4/r. Tel. No. 055 294 520 (between Via del Corso and Via delle Oche near the Duomo). Always remember that the plug adapter merely changes the configuration of the plug; it does not convert electricity.

Some problems have been reported by Americans using such chargers (bought in America) in Italy, even though the charger was switched to a 220-volt setting. If you experience problems, try plugging the charger into different wall outlets in the room. If the problem persists, you may want to rent an Italian charger.

Emergency Numbers

Emergency numbers to call for an ambulance or for a medical emergency (118), the carabinieri (112), the polizia (113), and the fire department (115) respond twenty-four hours a day and can also be dialed from a public phone without using coins or a card to pay for the call. You do not use an area code to call these numbers.

- **Ambulance** and medical emergencies: 118
- **Automobile Breakdown, ACI** (Italian Automobile Association): 803 116
- **Carabinieri** (Military Police): 112
- **Comando Provinciale Carabinieri:** Borgo Ognissanti, 48, Tel. No. 055 24 811. Open twenty-four hours a day. To report theft, lost property, missing persons. Useful when the Tourist Aid Police Office is closed.

- **Fire Department** (Vigili del Fuoco): 115
- **Polizia** (State Police): 113
- **Questura:** Via Zara, 2. Tel. No. 055 49 771. Open twenty-four hours. To report theft, lost property, missing persons. Office to report lost property is open from 8:30 to 20:00.
- **Tourist Aid Police:** Via Pietrapiana, 50 (near Piazza dei Ciompi). Tel. No. 055 203 911; Fax 055 2039 1379. Open Monday-Friday, 8:30-19:30; Saturday, 8:30-13:30. To report stolen or lost property. Interpreters available.
- **Towed cars:** Tel. No. 055 308 249. Even if your car has been towed, if you have left your disability parking permit on the dashboard, chances are that the car has simply been moved nearby and not towed to a city lot far away. Thus, while you might be charged a fine for the infraction, you will not have to pay for the tow fee nor suffer the consequences of having to go pick up your towed car. Infractions include parking on a crosswalk, at a bus stop, in a reserved parking place unless specifically designated by a (unnumbered) disability sign, in front of a *passo carrabile* (keep entrance clear) sign. If you cannot find your car, call the number given above, and if it has been moved, they will be able to tell you where it is.
- **Vigili urbani:** (Municipal Police) Main office in Porta a Prato, 6, Tel. No. 055 32 831. Twenty-four-hour call number: 055 328 3333.

Equipment Rental and Repair

- **Amplifon**, Piazza della Repubblica, 3. Tel. No. 055 210 069 or 283 823. Sells and repairs hearing devices. Not wheelchair accessible.
- **Gualtieri** has two stores: in Via T. Alderotti, 67 (near the Careggi Hospital). Designated parking space in front of store. One step up onto sidewalk. One step (9.5 centimeters [3 ¾ inches]) at entrance. Tel. No. 055 436 0386; Fax:

055 419 826; and in Viale Europa, 63 (south Florence). Tel/Fax: 055 683 634; home page: *www.gualtieri.it*; E-mail: *info@gualtieri.it*. Rental of manual wheelchairs, crutches, hospital beds. Will deliver. English spoken. Repairs are done in Via delle Panche, 56, Tel. No. 055 434 666.

- **Ortopedia Giotto**, Via del Romito 57/c. Tel. No. 055 463 3154; Fax: 055 463 2397. Home page: *www.barbieriweb.it*. E-mail: *giotto@katamail.com*. Rental and repair. Will pick up and deliver for both rentals and repair.
- **Ortopedia Paoletti**, Via Scipione Ammirato. Tel. No. 055 677 007. Closed on Saturday. Home page: *www. ortopediapaoletti.it*. E-mail: *paoletti@fibcc.it*. Rental of manual wheelchairs. Will deliver.

Getting Oriented

Layout of the City

Florence is divided roughly in half by the Arno river running from east to west. The oldest and main part of the *centro storico* or historic center lies north of the river where many of the city's most important monuments are located including the cathedral or Duomo; the Baptistery, Palazzo Vecchio, and the Uffizi Museum. Piazza della Repubblica, the main city square, Piazza del Duomo and Piazza della Signoria, together with surrounding streets, are pedestrian areas, closed to major traffic with the exception of police cars, taxis, and electric city buses. In addition, many of the sidewalks in this part of town have recently been rebuilt with smoother stone surfaces and curb cuts.

In the Middle Ages, Florence expanded to the south side of the river which eventually became known as the "Oltrarno" or "other side of the Arno." With few exceptions, such as Via Maggio or Via Guicciardini, most streets and sidewalks on the south side of the river are quite narrow and a useful aid to getting around if you are mobility impaired is the city accessibility map (see "Florence" in the chapter on "Resources").

For easy orientation in walking around the city, just remember that the Duomo lies on the north bank of the Arno, while San Miniato and Piazzale Michelangelo are on the south bank. Ponte alle Grazie is upstream towards the east, Ponte alla Carraia and the Cascine Park are downstream to the west.

Street Numbering

Following a general European rule of thumb, the sequence of Florentine street numbers is determined by an important geographical or urban feature such as the river or a city square. Lower numbers begin at the source (the Arno or Piazza della Repubblica) and increase as you move further away from it. Even numbers are on the right; uneven numbers on the left.

Two sets of numbers can be used on any given street, indicated by the colors red and black. Red numbers, always designated by a red *r*, indicate a commercial address; black numbers are usually used for a residence or a hotel. Note: Red numbers will always designate a commercial property, but not all commercial properties use red numbers.

Health

Ambulance Service

- **Misericordia** in Piazza del Duomo, 19/20, Tel. No. 055 212 222. Small donation requested.

Laboratory Analysis

- **Istituto Prosperius** in Via Fratelli Rosselli, 60/62, Tel. No. 055 238 1634. E-mail: *prosperius@prosperius.it*. Wheelchair-accessible entrance is from the parking lot.
- **Istituto Fanfani** in Piazza dell'Indipendenza, 18/b. Tel. No. 055 49 701; Fax: 055 497 0284. Home page: *www.istitutofanfani.it*. E-mail: *info@istitutofanfani.it*. Ramp at main entrance.

Medical Assistance: Nurses, Personal Care Attendants, and Travel Companions

- **Cooperativa Il Girasole** (Viale Talenti, 160, Florence. Tel/Fax: 055 739 9201. Home Page: *www.coopilgirasole.it*; e-mail: *segreteria@coopilgirasole.it*. Can provide a nurse, a personal care attendant, or travel companion during your stay in Florence. Hourly rates are €20,00 for medical assistance, €14,00 for attendant or companion service. It is best to contact them first by written request either by fax or e-mail.

Medical Insurance

- Italian citizens and members of the European Union are covered by the Italian National Health Care Program. Everyone else must pay for emergency room services and hospitalization. If you are not a member of the European Union, carrying a medical insurance policy with coverage abroad is essential.

Medical Service with English-Speaking Doctors

- **Ambulatorio della Misericordia** (near Piazza del Duomo in Vicolo degli Adimari, 1, Tel. No. 055 212 221) is a medical clinic for tourists with English-speaking doctors open Monday-Friday, 14:00-17:00. Small fee. No appointment necessary. A more extensive service with specialists is available at the clinic Monday-Friday, 8:00-20:00, and on Saturday, 8:00-13:00 by appointment only. The clinic, which is located upstairs, is reached by a wheelchair-accessible elevator (door width: 75 centimeters [29 ½ inches]; cabin length: 125 centimeters [just under 49 ¼ inches]) and has a wheelchair-accessible restroom.
- **Dr. Stephen Kerr** is an English general practitioner living in Florence with an office around the corner from the Molteni Pharmacy in Piazza della Signoria. The office is in

Via Porta Rossa, 1, located on the second floor and is not wheelchair accessible. However, Dr. Kerr is available for consultation by phone: office 055 288 055 or mobile phone 335 8361682, and his useful web site offers some interesting information about medical service in Florence: *www.dr-kerr.com*

- **Tourist Medical Center** (Studio Medico Associato in Via Lorenzo il Magnifico, 59, Tel. No. 055 475 411) is a private medical service open twenty-four hours with eight English— and French-speaking doctors. Office visits are without appointment, Monday-Saturday, 11:00-12:00; Monday-Friday, 17:00-18:00. Cost € 45,00. The office is not accessible to wheelchairs: six steps at main entrance; no accessible restroom. House calls can be made by appointment on weekdays, Sundays, and holidays by calling the above number. If the office is closed, leave a message, and you will be contacted within an hour. Cost of a house call is between €65,00 and €130,00.

Medical Translators

- **AVO** (Associazione Volontari Ospedalieri) Via Carducci, 4, Tel. No. 055 234 4567 or 055 425 0126. The Association of Hospital Volunteers has a group of interpreters who assist patients in communicating with doctors and hospital staff.

Public Hospitals and Hospitalization

The emergency room of the hospital is called the *pronto soccorso*. Any foreigner who is not a member of the European Union is expected to pay both for emergency room treatment and for hospitalization. If you are hospitalized, you must supply your own flatware, glass and dishes, towels, soap, and toilet paper. Bed linen is provided by the hospital. The following is a list of major public hospitals.

- **Arcispedale di Santa Maria Novella** in Piazza Santa Maria Novella, 1, closest to the historic center. Tel. No. 055 27 581.

- **Centro Traumatologico Ortopedico** (known as "CTO"), the city's main orthopedic hospital in Largo P. Palagi, 1. Tel. No. 055 427 8360.
- **Nuovo Ospedale di San Giovanni di Dio** in Via Torregalli, 3, at Scandicci (FI), a small general hospital located on the outskirts of Florence. Tel. No. 055 71 921.
- **Ospedale Anna Meyer** in Via L. Giordano, 13, the children's hospital. Tel. No. 055 56 621.
- **Ospedale Oftalmico Fiorentino** in Via Pico della Mirandola, the ophthalmic hospital. Tel. No. 055 56 621.
- **Ospedale Santa Maria Annunziata** in Via dell'Antella at Antella, small general hospital located on the outskirts of Florence. Tel. No. 055 24 961. The **dialysis center** is open to tourists, but appointments must be scheduled at least one month in advance. Tel. No. 055 249 6520 for information and appointments. Requests can be made by fax by contacting the Centro Dialisi at Tel. No. 055 249 6671.
- **Policlinico di Careggi** in Viale Morgagni, 85, the city's teaching hospital connected with the University of Florence. Tel. No. 055 427 7111. The CTO (see above) is part of this hospital.

Pharmacies

American prescriptions are not considered valid and will have to be rewritten by a doctor who is licensed to practice in Italy. Many medicines and drugs are now also labeled in Braille. While each chapter contains a brief list of wheelchair-accessible pharmacies in a specific neighborhood, the following is a list of **twenty-four-hour pharmacies** which are also open on Sunday.

- **Farmacia all'Insegna del Moro** in Piazza San Giovanni, 20/r, near the Duomo and Baptistery. Tel. No. 055 211 343.
- **Farmacia Comunale, 13,** located inside the Station of Santa Maria Novella. Tel. No. 055 216 761.
- **Farmacia Molteni** in Via Calzaiuoli, 7/r, just off Piazza della Signoria. Tel. No. 055 289 490 or 215 472.

Physical Therapy

- **Istituto Prosperius** in Via Masaccio, 127. Tel. No. 055 500 1465.

Holidays and Local Celebrations

During the following holidays, banks, offices, schools, shops, and for the more standard holidays, many museums are closed: New Year's Day, January 6 (Epiphany), April 25 (Liberation Day), Easter and Easter Monday, May 1 (Labor Day), June 24 (only in Florence: feast day of the city's patron, St. John the Baptist), August 15 (Assumption of the Virgin), November 1 (All Saint's Day), December 8 (Immaculate Conception), Christmas, and December 26 (St. Stephen's Day).

Some colorful local celebrations of special interest are described below:

- The **Scoppio del Carro,** a festival whose origins date to the First Crusade, takes place on Easter morning. A festive towering cart, drawn through the streets by white oxen, is positioned in front of the Duomo, and at the conclusion of mass, the archbishop ignites a mechanical dove which flies from the high altar on a steel wire to the cart to set off fireworks.
- **La Festa del Grillo** takes place in May on Ascension Day when children are taken to the Cascine Park to buy crickets in wooden cages.
- In June a series of three **Calcio in Costume** or soccer games in historic costume commemorate an event of 1530 when the Florentines chose to play soccer in defiance of the Spanish and papal troops that held the city under siege. The final game is played on June 24 to celebrate St. John's Feast Day, followed by a spectacular fireworks display in the evening from Piazzale Michelangelo.

- In early September, during the **Festa delle Rificolone**, children carry lighted paper lanterns through the streets to celebrate the birth date of the Virgin.

Local Customs and Etiquette

Calling a cab and hailing a bus. It is difficult to hail a cab in Florence where taxis generally do not "cruise" but park in designated taxi stands. For location of taxi stands and for telephone numbers, see the chapter on "Transportation." Instead, if you are waiting for a bus, make sure to hail it, otherwise it may just keep on going. The reason for this is that several differently routed buses may use the same stop.

Distinguishing the floors of a building. The ground floor is always referred to as the *piano terra* or *pianterreno,* marked "PT," "T," or "0" in an elevator. The first floor, known as the *primo piano* or sometimes the *piano nobile* corresponds to the first floor above ground (actually the American second floor) and will be marked "1" in the elevator. Therefore, if your hotel room is on the *quarto piano* (the "fourth floor"), it's actually on the fifth floor.

Dress codes. Florentines tend to dress more formally than many tourists. With the exception of the younger crowd, many of them do not wear summer shorts in the center of town. Churches can be very strict on dress, sometimes refusing entry if you are wearing shorts or have bare upper arms. Some of the more important churches such as the Duomo will lend you a "cover-up" in case you should forget.

Salutations. The *ciao* that you so often hear for saying both "hi" or "good-bye" is used exclusively between friends. Although their attitude is open and friendly, Italians, and especially Florentines who are more reserved than southern Italians, always speak to strangers or mere acquaintances more formally. Therefore, when you enter a store, a restaurant, or go to breakfast in your hotel, the phrase to use in the morning is *buon giorno*. You can also use the same phrase to say "good-bye" when you leave. Right after lunch, from early afternoon into the evening, the greeting used in Florence is *buona sera* (literally "good evening"). However, in almost all other parts of Italy, you will continue to use *buon giorno* throughout the afternoon. *Buona notte* ("good night") is used in late-night situations, for instance, upon leaving a restaurant after dinner. On reentering your hotel, first greet the concierge with *buona sera*. After collecting the key, say *buona notte* as you go up to your room to bed. The phrase *arrivederci,* although less formal, is still acceptable upon leaving a taxi, a restaurant, or a store, but don't be surprised if you are answered with the more formal *arrivederla*.

Telling time. Official time schedules for trains and planes, opening hours of banks, offices, shops, restaurants, or museums, the hours of a theatrical performance or film will always be expressed according to the European twenty-four-hour system. For example, 1 p.m. American time is 13:00, 3 p.m. is 15:00, and 24:00 is midnight. Only in casual conversation will you hear someone refer to "3 o'clock in the afternoon" (le 3 [tre] del pomeriggio). To avoid confusion, opening times indicated in this guidebook follow the twenty-four-hour system.

Tipping. Rules for tipping are complicated, but in general, Italians either don't tip at all or else token tip if service is good. Because American tourists usually tip out of habit, they are, unfortunately, often expected to do so, but stick to your guns if you feel that the service does not deserve a tip. For a taxi ride, 10 percent is generous, but you may want to offer this if you've been given extra assistance. It's also permissible to round off and up to the nearest 0,50 cents which is what many Italians do. In restaurants a 15 percent service charge is automatically included in the final bill indicated by the words *servizio compreso* or *servizio incluso* on the bill. Always ask if you are uncertain. It is still customary to leave a little something on top of this, bringing the service charge up to a total of 17 or 18 percent. If you want to leave more, underpaid waiters are always grateful for a generous tip especially if they've given you good service. Sometimes restroom attendants will charge a set fee (around 0,60 cents) or expect a similar amount in exchange for soap, towels, or toilet paper.

Opening Hours

Many stores, banks, offices, and pharmacies are closed in the middle of the day, and their opening hours may sometimes vary according to season. In August, when most Italians are away on vacation, many theaters and indoor cinemas, restaurants and stores, especially those located outside the immediate center of town, may close either for all or for part of the month.

- **Banks** are open Monday through Friday, 8:30-13:20 and 14:30-15:30. They are closed on Saturdays and Sundays. Depending on the bank, opening and closing times may vary slightly but usually no more than five or ten minutes.
- **Churches** are usually open from around 7:00-12:00 and 16:00-18:00, but depending on the individual church, these times may vary slightly. The cathedral or Duomo and the Basilica of Santa Croce are open all day but closed Sunday morning.
- **Museums** such as the Accademia, the Palazzo Vecchio, and the Uffizi, which are large and important, stay open all day. Smaller museums may close as early as 14:00.
- **Restaurants** are open between 12:45 and 15:00 for lunch; 19:45-22:30 for dinner although some may open earlier or close later. Most are usually closed one day a week.
- **Shops** have varying hours depending on their activity, but in general they are closed in the middle of the day. Food shops open around 8:00, close around 13:00 or 13:30 and then reopen 17:00-20:00 and, with few exceptions, are closed on Wednesday afternoon. Most other shops open around 9:00, while some clothing stores may not open until 10:00.

Except for the larger department stores, supermarkets, and some select stores in the historic center, they all close around 13:00 and reopen around 15:30-16:00 until 19:30-20:00. Many nonfood stores are closed Monday morning. During the summer months, all stores are likely to close also on Saturday afternoon and many sometime during the month of August.

Restrooms

Florence is generally short on public restrooms and especially on those which are accessible. Below you will find a list of public restrooms, including those located in two centrally located department stores which, unlike many places, are open all day, even on Monday morning when most stores and many museums are closed. In addition to this list, consult the chapters regarding the different geographical sections of the city where you will find a list of the accessible restrooms found in the museums, bars, restaurants, cafés, and hotels located in that specific neighborhood. Note: The word "accessible" in Italy is a term that is often tossed around lightly. Indications have been made when necessary to note the shortcomings of some situations. Descriptions regarding the location of grab bars and transfer space are given as if you were facing the WC. Public restrooms charge a small fee of €0,60 (about seventy cents). In 2003 public restrooms in the center of town and at Piazzale Michelangelo remained open until midnight in the months of August and September.

- **La Rinascente** department store (Piazza della Repubblica, 1; Tel. No. 055 219 113; hours: 9:00-21:00, Monday-Saturday; Sunday, 10:30-20:00.) With a 2.5-centimeter (1-inch) lip at front entrance. **Elevator** (depth: 150 centimeters [59 inches]) is also suitable for scooters. Restroom is located on the top floor on the southeast corner of the store in the household dept. Ask a salesperson for the key which is kept in the customer service office on the west side of the store opposite the elevator to the café upstairs. Restroom has horizontal and vertical grab bars to the right of the WC (height: 51 centimeters [20 inches]) with transfer space from left.

- **Coin** department store (Via Calzaiuoli, 56r; Tel. No. 055 280 531; hours: 9:30-20:00, Monday-Saturday; Sunday, 11:00-20:00). The restroom is located on the ground floor in the men's department in the section called "Coin Uomo" (from Via Calzaiuoli go straight towards the back of the store, turn left after the stairs). Ask a salesperson for the key. Restroom has vertical grab bars to right rear and left front of WC (height: 47 centimeters [18 ½ inches]); unwrapped metal pipe under sink.
- **Railroad station of Santa Maria Novella** located next to track 5. Small fee.
- **Near the San Lorenzo Market** in Via della Stufa, 25. Open 10:00-18:00; 9:00-19:00, June-September. Small fee. A heavy wooden ramp is placed on request in front of the door. Grab bars on right of WC; space for left transfer.
- **Near Santa Croce** at the tourist information office of the city of Florence in Borgo Santa Croce, 29/r; open Monday-Saturday, 9:00-19:00; Sunday, 9:00-14:00. Steep short slope at main entrance. Small fee.
- **Between Santa Croce and Piazza della Signoria** in Via Filippina, corner Via Borgognona. Open 9:00-18:00; 9:00-19:00, June-September. Ramp at entrance. Small fee.
- **Between Ponte Santa Trinita and Ponte Vecchio** in Via dello Sprone. Open 10:00-18:00; 9:00-19:00, June-September. Ramp at entrance. Small fee.
- **Near Piazzale Michelangelo.** Open 8:30-18:00, Monday-Saturday. Small fee (must purchase a ticket from the ticket machine located inside the restroom). Directions: Cross the street from the *piazzale* at the crosswalk in front of the two sidewalk café/bars and go 108 meters (354 feet) in the direction of Porta Romana and the Church of San Miniato.

The restroom is on your left beyond the ramp leading to the restaurant La Loggia.

- **In the Cascine Park** near Piazzale Kennedy at the center of the park. Open 10:00-17:00; 9:00-19:00, June-September. Small fee.

Reservations

- **Museums**
  Call **Firenze Musei**, Tel. No. 055 294 883, Monday-Friday, 8:30-18:30, and Saturday, 9:00-12:00 for reservations at state museums. For further details, see chapter on "Museums, Music, Movies, and Sports."

- **Concert Tickets**
  Box Office in Via Alamanni, 39 (near Station of Santa Maria Novella). Open 10:00-19:30 except Monday morning and Sunday. Tel. No. 055 210 804. There is a 15 percent markup for the reservation service on some tickets, but not for those of the Teatro Comunale. E-mail: *firenze@boxoffice.it*. Web site: *www.boxoffice.it*. Can reserve and pay by credit card online. There is a more centrally located branch office on the fourth floor of La Rinascente Department Store in Piazza della Repubblica.
  Teatro Comunale in Corso Italia, 16. Tel. No. 055 211 158. Ticket office open 10:00-18:00, on Saturday 10:00-13:00. Designated parking place outside box office. Or purchase online: *tickets@maggiofiorentino.com*. For season schedule: *www.maggiofiorentino.com*.

Sales Tax Refunds

Part of the tax you pay on purchases in European Union countries is called VAT (or "IVA" in Italian). By law all non-EU residents are entitled to a refund on purchases of €155,00 or over made at shops participating in the tax-free offer. Participating shops will usually display the *Tax-Free* Shopping sign. The refund can sometimes amount to as much as 20 percent of the cost of your purchase. On making your purchase, you fill out a tax-free card and will receive a document stating the amount of reimbursement. Before leaving the country, you must go to a Global Refund office with the document received from the store, the receipt, and the unused goods. Within three months, you will receive your refund. For further information see *www.globalrefund.com* or *www.e-shopagain.com.* E-mail: *taxfree@it.globalrefund.com.* Global Refund offices in Florence are located on the Ponte Vecchio, 2 (Tel. No. 055 211 567 or 217 046) and at the Amerigo Vespucci Airport at Peretola (055 302 4285 or 375 226). The Ponte Vecchio office is on the second floor (1° *piano*), and its tiny elevator is not accessible to wheelchairs. The airport office is located in the Departures Building.

Tourist Information Centers (opening times are subject to change)

- **Near Palazzo Medici: APT** (Azienda Promozionale Turistica/ Provincial Tourist Board Office), Via Cavour, 1/r. Tel. No. 055 290 832. Open Monday-Saturday, 8:30-18:30; Sundays, 8:30-13:30.
- **At the A. Vespucci airport** in the arrivals building: **APT** Tel. No. 055 315 874.
- **Across from the RR station: Ufficio Informazione Turistica** (Tourist Information Office of the city of Florence), Piazza Stazione, 4; Tel. No. 055 212 245. Open Monday-Friday, 8:30-19:00; Saturday-Sunday, 8:30-13:30. (There is a platform lift next to the staircase down to the information area, but few members of the staff seem to know how it works. No call bell.)
- **Near Church of Santa Croce: Ufficio Informazione Turistica** (Tourist Information Office of the city of Florence), Borgo Santa Croce, 29/r; Tel. No. 055 234 0444 or 055 226 4524. Open Monday-Saturday, 9:00-19:00; Sunday, 9:00-14:00 (has wheelchair-accessible restroom; small fee).

- **Tourist Help.** Two vans (with municipal police and APT representatives) are stationed in Piazza della Repubblica and at the foot of the Ponte Vecchio on the Oltrarno side to answer questions and to distribute informative material to tourists.

Veterinary Medical Service

- Dr. John Mucera, an American veterinarian, is available for house calls in and outside of Florence. Tel. No. 055 237 3120. Mobile phone: 347 4 620 710. E-mail: *Dvmoncall@hotmail.com.*

Contact for appointments and information about bringing domestic animals to Italy. Dr. Mucera collaborates with Dr. Fabio Fanfani at Dr. Fanfani's veterinary clinic "Certosa" (Via Senese, 286, Galluzzo (FI) Tel. No. 055 204 8338. Open Monday-Saturday, 9:00-13:00 and 16:00-20:00; Sunday, 11:00-13:00) where he can be found in the afternoons.

Transportation

Getting to Florence

By Train

The Italian Railway offers assistance free of charge to passengers travelling by medium or long distance trains to one hundred ninety-six different destinations located throughout the country; however, facilities on board can vary widely. The newer Eurostar trains have cars equipped with an adapted restroom and places for two wheelchairs and two companions. To request this service, call the "Centro di Accoglienza" (Customer Assistance Center) of the station where your trip originates at least twenty-four hours ahead of departure. Three working days advance notice is required for international journeys. The center will reserve a place for you on the train, help with boarding and luggage and, upon arrival, accompany you to the station's exit. A wheelchair can be provided for use in the station until you board. Boarding by wheelchair is done by platform lift.* Upon prior arrangement, the dining car can serve meals at your reserved seat. For a small fee the Customer Assistance Center can mail your ticket to your place of residence, or you can arrange to pick the ticket up directly at the Customer Assistance Center.

In making your request, be as specific as possible about the kind of assistance you need: if you will require help boarding the train, in changing trains, will need to borrow a wheelchair, order from the dining car, or require assistance at your destination. Be sure to arrive at the station at least forty-five minutes before time of departure.

If you are arriving in Florence from Rome, the arrangements for your trip to Florence will be made in Rome. Call 06 488 1726 for departures from both Rome's Termini RR station or from the Leonardo da Vinci airport at Fiumicino. Numbers for Customer Assistance Centers in major cities are Bologna: 051 630 3132; Florence: 055 235 2275; Genoa: 010 274 3775; Milan: 02 6707 0958; Naples: 081 567 2991; Turin: 011 669 0447; Venice: 041 785 570. (Remember to add international access code and country code [39] when dialing from outside Italy.)

For departures from Florence's main railway station of Santa Maria Novella, the "Centro di Accoglienza" is located next to track 5. The station's adapted restroom is located at the top of track 5, and lowered telephones are situated throughout the station. **Wheelchair access to the station is from the main "Arrivals" entrance or by a small ramp at the taxi stand nearby. There is a high curb at the "Departures" entrance.**

For further information, a complete list of Customer Assistance Centers, train schedules, and purchase of tickets online see *www.trenitalia.com.* For specific information regarding the "Centri di Accoglienza" click on "servizi per i disabili." (Accessibility information is given in Italian only.)

*Important: The railroad specifically states that this service is available for users of manual wheelchairs. If you are travelling by electric scooter or by large power wheelchair, although with some persuasion the Customer Assistance Center will usually comply with your request, they are not under obligation to do so according to their standard policy. Make sure to give the dimensions of the scooter or power chair in order to allow the railroad personnel to determine whether it will fit on the platform lift and in the train. In special circumstances such as this, make plans well in advance.

By Plane

Florence's **"Amerigo Vespucci" airport**, located approximately five kilometers northwest of the city's center, serves a number of

Italian domestic and European destinations. While there are no direct flights to the USA, connecting flights can be arranged via various cities including Rome, Milan, Amsterdam, Brussels, London, Paris, Frankfort, Munich, and Zurich.

Both arrivals and departures terminals are equipped with accessible restrooms and elevators to the upper-level coffee bars and restaurants. Lift buses are used to board the planes. An accessible parking space, equipped with phone to call for assistance with baggage, is located in front of the "Departures" building. Several designated accessible parking spaces are located in a small area just in front of the "Arrivals" building. Twelve designated accessible parking spaces are found in the airport parking lot for which no fee is charged if you show your permit (American permits are accepted).

The Florence airport has no jet ways, and passengers are taken to the plane by bus and then board the plane by stairs. Boarding vehicles with lifts are used to board passengers in wheelchairs or those passengers who cannot walk up the stairs to the plane. If you use a wheelchair, when you check in, make sure to request a seat at the front of the plane since there is usually less room to board through the rear door. The staff may try to insist that you transfer to an airport manual wheelchair in order to load yours onto the plane, transferring you to a narrower aisle chair when it is time to board. Stick to your guns if you do not wish to make the intermediate transfer. Many of the airport staff have not been properly trained to deal with people travelling in wheelchairs and do not understand that, for some people, transferring can be difficult. Among other problems encountered at the Florence airport: One passenger was recently boarded on an aisle chair that was not padded, had no arm rests, and only one seat belt, instead of the customary three.

Presently no accessible bus lines serve the Florence airport, and transportation to and from the center of town is usually by taxi. For information on reserving a wheelchair-accessible cab or private van, see below. For detailed information on the airport's general services see *www.safnet.it* (click on "passenger service," then "special assistance").

While not as convenient as flying into Florence, both Pisa's "Galileo Galilei" and Bologna's "G. Marconi" airports are about an hour's distance away. Train service to Florence directly from the Pisa airport is accessible to wheelchair users even though the airport trains are not equipped with designated seating or tie downs. Pisa's central railway station is located less than a mile away with wheelchair-accessible trains leaving for Florence approximately every hour. Another option to get to Florence from the Pisa Airport is to hire an accessible private van or accessible cab from Florence (see below) For information on the Pisa's airport's services: *www.pisa-airport.com* (click on "enter," then "passenger services" and "services for the disabled").

Bologna's central railway station, located less than four miles (6 kilometers) from the airport, is frequently served by accessible Intercity and Eurostar trains. The COTABO cab company (Tel. No. 051 372 727) has accessible vehicles available. For reservations call 051 374 300. For information on the services offered by the Bologna airport see *www.bologna-airport.it* (click on "passenger services," then "disabled people").

By Automobile

Florence is easily reached via major multilane toll expressways or "autostrade": the A1 from Naples to Rome, Florence, Bologna, and Milan and the A11 from Florence to Lucca and Pisa. Almost all service areas on these roads are equipped with accessible restrooms. There are no service areas on the four-lane, toll-free "superstrada" from Florence to Siena except for two new service areas with accessible restrooms (one on each side of the highway) at the Siena end. The toll-free "superstrada" Florence-Pisa-Livorno has a service area with accessible restroom at "Pontedera nord" (direction Pisa).

Important note: While gas stations are open throughout the day on the autostrada and superstrada with self-service pumps open at night, most other gas stations both in the cities and on other major highways close at night around 19:00 (7 p.m.); in the middle of the day (usually between 12:30 and 15:30); often on Saturday afternoons and on Sundays. Not all stations have self-service pumps.

Getting Around

Driving

Between 7:30 a.m. and 7:30 p.m., Monday through Saturday, Florence's historic center, known as the *zona blu* or ZTL (Limited Traffic Zone), is closed to normal traffic. Holders of disability parking permits, however, are allowed to enter the *zona blu* and are also permitted to drive in all areas otherwise limited to taxis, buses, police, ambulances, and pedestrians.

According to a resolution reached in 1997 by the European Conference of Ministers of Transportation (ECMT), both EU members and, by special agreement, citizens of the United States, Australia, Japan, Korea, New Zealand, and Canada in possession of disability parking permits, can use their permit in EU countries. Therefore, American disability parking permits are considered valid in Italy.

Obtaining permission to drive in Florence has become more complicated since the recent introduction of a new system of controlling access to the ZTL by electronic eye camera. Resident drivers with permits who are allowed to circulate in the ZTL must now, in addition to displaying their permit on the dashboard of their car, obtain a "Telepass" or electronic beeper device which must be fixed to the windshield of their car. Visitors to Florence who possess disability parking permits are still entitled to enter the ZTL but must communicate this information to the proper authorities and either be placed on a special exemption list or obtain a temporary "Telepass."

If you plan to drive in Florence and are staying in a hotel located within the ZTL, be sure to alert the hotel that you are driving a car. It is up to the hotel to contact the proper authorities who will then place you on the exemption list (called the *lista bianca*). If you are not staying in a hotel in the center of Florence and still plan to enter the ZTL, you can stop by any municipal police office to ask to be inserted on the list. Requests can be made Monday-Friday only, but you are allowed to make this request even on the day after you enter the ZTL. (If you enter on a Friday, you have until the following Monday to communicate your information.) The main municipal police office is located at Porta a Prato, 6. Tel. No. 055 32 831. Other convenient police offices are located just inside of Porta Romana in Piazza della Calza, 2 (Tel. No. 055 221 001) and inside the Palazzo Vecchio (Tel. No. 055 284 926). An alternative is to communicate your information directly by fax to the Consulta Invalidi di Firenze (Town Council on Disability Issues) Tel. No./Fax: 055 321 5145. Be sure your request includes a photocopy of your permit, when and where the permit was issued, the dates and time you wish to enter the ZTL, and your car license number. This information must be communicated every time you wish to enter the limited traffic zone. If you are planning to stay in Florence for a long period, you will need to obtain a temporary "Telepass" beeper. To obtain this, you must go the office of Firenze Parcheggi, Viale Matteotti 50/A (Tel. No. 055 503 021). Open Monday-Friday, 8:30-13:00 and 14:00-16:30. The office is wheelchair accessible. You will be required to leave a €48,00 deposit, to be refunded when you return the "Telepass" at the end of your visit.

Parking

Because of limited circulation, designated accessible parking spaces within the historic center's ZTL are scarce. The *Mappa dell'Accessibilità Urbana* gives information on their location, but since the map was published in 2000, this information is sometimes out of date. The publication *The Florence Experience* provides more recent information, but some of the parking spaces mentioned in the book are not always clearly indicated on the street.

Reserved parking spaces should always be designated with an

orange international disability symbol displayed on a vertical signpost or marked in orange (sometimes in blue) directly on the pavement. If a signpost should carry a symbol with a number under it, do not park there; this is a reserved space for a disabled resident.

According to the 1997 ECMT ruling mentioned above, holders of disability parking permits in any EU member country and in the United States and Canada are entitled to the same parking privileges allowed to permit holders in Italy. Permit holders are allowed to park without paying on streets where there is a pay meter or "pay and display" parking, as well as in public parking lots. All public parking lots have designated parking spaces for those in possession of disability parking permits. Public lots with fifty or fewer places are required to have at least one designated parking space, and if this is occupied, you are still entitled to park without paying even if you occupy another space. Private parking lots are not required to follow the same regulations. For further information on the ECMT ruling and for specifics on disability parking in Italy, see *www.oecd.org/cem/topics/handicaps/parking.htm.*

By tacit agreement, disability parking permit holders who have received permission to enter the ZTL are allowed to park inside the chained-off area behind the Duomo, in Piazza della Signoria on the north side of Palazzo Vecchio opposite the wheelchair-accessible entrance, in Piazza Santa Croce near Via Verdi, and on the north and south edges of Piazza della Repubblica, even though these parking spaces are not marked.

Convenient, centrally located, twenty-four-hour parking with a reserved, accessible parking area is located under the Station of Santa Maria Novella. This parking lot is about ten minutes from Piazza del Duomo. It is permitted to reach the parking lot, which is in the ZTL, only by taking Via S. Caterina d'Alessandria, then Via Nazionale, from Viale Lavagnini or Via Diacceto, then Via Alamanni, from Viale Rosselli. To park in the area reserved for those who possess disability parking permits, it's best to enter the garage from the Piazza della Stazione. At the first barrier gate inside the parking garage, stop and take ticket. Straight ahead is a second barrier gate at the entrance to the reserved area. The second barrier gate is electronically connected to the office upstairs. Ring and the gate should then raise automatically. If you are asked for identification, say that you have a disability parking permit (*Ho un contrassegno per disabili*). You can also park in any other available space in the garage, but free spaces are sometimes difficult to find when the garage is full. Be sure to show your permit at the cash register upstairs when you are ready to leave. You will be given a ticket to insert into the barrier gate when you exit from the garage. Parking for those with disability parking permits is free.

For those exiting from the Autostrada A1 at "Firenze-Certosa" or coming to Florence from Siena who do not want to deal with city traffic, three parking lots are located on the south side of the city. One of these lots is located about a half kilometer outside Porta Romana in Via del Gelsomino (with accessible restroom; parking lot attendant has key). Wheelchair-accessible Bus No. 11 stops nearby in Via del Gelsomino, or you can ask the parking attendant to call a taxi to take you into town. The other two parking lots are located nearer to town next to the medieval city gate of Porta Romana: one to the right as you face the city gate from Piazzale Porta Romana (one reserved space); the other to the left just inside the city gate in Piazza la Calza with two reserved parking spaces near the entrance on the left. Entrance to the parking lot is under the far-left arch of the gate. Outside the gate in Piazzale Porta Romana are a taxi stand and two bus stops: one for wheelchair-accessible Bus No. 13 (direction Station of Santa Maria Novella) to the left of the gate in Viale Petrarca, the other for wheelchair-accessible Bus No. 12 (direction Piazzale Michelangelo) opposite the gate in Piazzale Porta Romana.

Taxis

If you are able to transfer to a seat, many regular taxis are station wagons, and drivers are usually helpful in giving assistance. A small tip (for assistance with baggage or wheelchair) is accepted willingly.

Presently Florence has four accessible taxis: two equipped with ramps, two with lifts. One taxi with lift circulates freely; the other three taxis remain in the garage unless specifically requested. All four can be reserved for railway and airport arrivals and departures (including the airports of Florence, Bologna, and Pisa), for normal service within the city, or for half—or full-day excursions outside Florence. In all cases, it is best to call in advance. To reserve an accessible taxi, call the COTAFI cab company at 055 4390 or 055 4499 (Fax: 055 419 829; E-mail: *taxi4390@tin.it*). This company has one FIAT Scudo taxi with lift, holding four passengers and one wheelchair; maximum head clearance is 128 centimeters (50 $^3/8$ inches) to enter; 136 centimeters (53 ½ inches) inside the cab. Their approximate fares are €25,00 for the Florence airport (if the plane is on time and the taxi is not required to wait); €150,00 for the Pisa airport; €200,00 for the Bologna airport (add 10 percent tax to quoted price). The SOCOTA cab company at 055 4242 or 055 4798 has one taxi with lift and two others with ramps. All three of their Volkswagon taxis hold seven passengers and one wheelchair and have a maximum head clearance of 130 centimeters (51 3/16 inches).

You do not hail a cab in Florence but either call one of the numbers given above (explain that you are in a wheelchair to avoid getting a small car or a van-type vehicle with a high step) or go directly to a taxi stand. Some major stands in or near the center of town are located at the Station of Santa Maria Novella, in Piazza S. Marco, Piazza della Repubblica, Piazza Duomo (behind the cathedral), Piazza Santa Croce, and outside Porta Romana.

Buses

For details, also in English, of bus routes, schedules, and fares see *www.ataf.net*. Lines 7, 8, 12, 13, 20, 22, 23, 27, 29, 30, 31, 32, 33, 57, and D provide a 100 percent service of accessible buses* equipped with ramp and place for one wheelchair. Of special interests to tourists are the No. 7 (from the Santa Maria Novella RR station to Piazza San Marco and Fiesole), the No. 12 and No.

13 (clockwise and counterclockwise routes from the station to the Church of San Miniato and Piazzale Michelangelo), the No. 23 (from the station to the Duomo and Palazzo Vecchio, with return route past Santa Croce), and the D (from the station to the Ponte Vecchio, Palazzo Pitti, and Churches of Santo Spirito and the Carmine). Bus No. 8 goes to the hospital at Careggi; Bus No. 20 (direction "Gignoro") stops near the Cenacolo di San Salvi; Buses Nos. 31-32 (Grassina/Antella) stop near the Hospital of Santa Maria Annunziata.

*Warning: While the bus company tries to guarantee 100 percent service on accessible bus lines, once in a while you may find a nonaccessible bus. If so, just wait for the next one. The bus company has tried its best to provide satisfactory service, but they are unable to prevent unforeseen difficulties created by illegally parked vehicles which sometimes make it impossible to open the ramp properly. Sometimes the height of the sidewalk or lack of a properly elevated sidewalk on which to rest the ramp make descent and ascent dangerous, impossible or, at best, extremely difficult even with assistance. Not all bus stops are accessible, and it is best to ask the driver before you board if you will be able to get off the bus at your destination. It is advisable to travel always with a companion, even though many of the bus drivers are extremely courteous and willing to help.

- **Instructions for Using the Bus.** Always hail a bus as you would a cab, otherwise the bus you want may not stop. Instructions for wheelchair users: the newer buses have instructions in English, the older ones do not. All you need to know is that the **green button** blocks the wheels; the **blue button** disengages them. The **yellow button** requests a stop, the **red button** requests assistance. All buses are equipped with a safety belt. Remember the gradient of the ramp will depend on the height of the sidewalk. Also note, the threshold is sometimes tricky to maneuver (this is the point where the ramp slides out from under the floor of the bus). Maximum weight capacity of the ramps is 300 kilograms (660 pounds).

- **Bus Fares.** Tickets can be purchased at most bars, *tabaccherie* (tobacco shops), and many newsstands, and if you are planning to use the bus frequently, special fares can be purchased at the ATAF ticket office located opposite the "Arrivals" side of the Station of Santa Maria Novella. These include unlimited rides for twenty-four hours, two days, three days, seven days, and one month (riding the bus without a ticket is illegal and subject to a fine). For an idea of price: a ticket for a single ride valid for sixty minutes is €1, a thirty-day pass is €31,00. Tickets cannot be purchased on board the bus except between 9 p.m. and 6 a.m. Children under one meter in height (39.37 inches) travel free.

- **Electric Buses.** Of special interest to slow walkers are the small electric buses on lines A, B, C that crisscross the heart of the historic center. These buses are small, silent, and relatively easy to board. They are not accessible to wheelchairs and, if they do not approach a sidewalk, have a 29-centimeter (just under 11 ½-inch) step. Bus A leaves from the Santa Maria Novella RR station, going right through the center of Florence, passing Via Tornabuoni, Piazza della Repubblica, Orsanmichele, the Casa di Dante, Bargello Museum, and flea market in Piazza Ciompi before arriving in Piazza Beccaria. Bus B runs along the Arno, between Ponte della Vittoria and Ponte San Niccolò and passes by the Uffizi. Bus C connects Piazza San Marco to the section of the Oltrarno west of the Ponte Vecchio. Important stops along this route include Piazza San Marco, Piazza SS Annunziata, the Archaeological Museum, the Sant'Ambrogio Market, and Santa Croce. The buses run approximately every ten minutes between 8 a.m. and 8 p.m., but not on holidays or Sundays. Although free for residents, nonresidents must pay. If you plan to use them often, you can buy a special, thirty-day pass valid for buses A, B, C, D for about €14,50.

Car Rental

Presently, cars fitted with hand controls (usually Opel station wagons) are available for rent in Italy through Hertz. For reservations, call the Hertz Reservation Center at 199 112 211 (from Italy) or +39 02 694 3006 (from outside of Italy) at least seventy-two hours in advance. At the time of consignment, a document stating the driver's disability, together with driver's license, must be presented. Although the cars are available in Rome and Milan, for an extra fee they can be picked up or dropped off at any Hertz office in Italy, including Florence. Hertz offices in Florence are located at the airport arrivals terminal (Tel. No. 055 307 370), near the station (Via Maso Finiguerra, 33, Tel. No. 055 239 8205), and near the autostrada (Via Novoli, 75, Tel. No. 055 436 2560).

Wheelchair-accessible Vans with Driver

There are several possibilities of hiring wheelchair-accessible vans with drivers for airport or station transfers and day trips. Prices run approximately between €35,00 to €40,00 for a transfer from the RR station to a hotel in town; €50,00 for an airport transfer; €160,00 to €200,00 for a half-day excursion to Siena; €160,00 to €190,00 for a transfer from the Pisa airport to Florence (add 10 percent tax to all quoted prices). Prices vary from company to company, and it pays to shop around.

- **Co.A.Ve** (Consorzio di Autoservizi "Amerigo Vespucci") in Florence (Via Giacomini, 28; 50132 Florence; Tel. No. 055 583 100; Fax: 055 553 2667; E-mail *coave@mail.dada.it*) has four adapted vans with ramp. The two smaller vans hold seven passengers and one wheelchair; the two larger vans, fourteen passengers and two wheelchairs. The vans can also carry four-wheel scooters.
- **SEFIR** in Florence (Via Paisiello, 11/r; 50144 Florence; Tel. No. 055 360 030; Fax: 055 332 088; E-mail

sefirsrl@tin.it) has a FIAT Ducato minibus with ramp and room for seven passengers and one wheelchair; head clearance 180 centimeters (just under 71 inches); and an IVECO Sitcar bus able to carry one wheelchair and twenty-eight passengers. A Mercedes Sprinter van (two wheelchairs; five passengers) is also available for hire on weekends, holidays, and during summer months.

* **MarcoViaggi** near Livorno (Via Genova, 20; Interno B/8; Località la Chiusa; 57014 Collesalvetti (Li); Tel/Fax: 0586 965 030; E-mail *marcoviaggi@infinito.it*) has three adapted vans available. One van with powered lift carries six passengers and one wheelchair. Two vans with powered ramp carry six passengers and two wheelchairs. This company is a good option for travelers arriving at the Pisa airport or on a cruise ship at Livorno. They also work in Florence.

Electric Vehicles

Slow walkers might consider hiring a small electric "golf carts" holding a maximum of four people available from "Biancaneve" autonoleggio rent car/vetture elettriche (Via Lulli, 62, Florence; mobile phone: 339 871 9125 or 339 332 6010; fax: 055 331 304; website: *www.biancaneve.org*). Because they run on electricity, these carts can be driven within most of Florence's historic center. Rates run around €17,00 for the first three hours and €55,00 per day. Special rates are available for longer rentals.

Accommodations

Sleeping in Florence is generally not cheap, but prices can range anywhere from a top-scale luxury hotel at around €700,00 or more a night to rock-bottom prices in a youth hostel where you might pay as little as €20,00, and there is a vast range in between. Accommodations in Florence, as elsewhere in Italy, are rated according to stars or *stelle*. Five-star luxury is at the top of the line; one star, on the budget end. While the number of stars will give you some indication of the price and the amenities included, they will not necessarily give you any indication of the atmosphere, and sometimes a two—or three-star hotel can offer a lot more charm than a higher-priced one.

There are a number of options of different types of places to stay in and around Florence. Aside from the standard hotel category, an increasing number of self-catering apartments are appearing on the market for those who are looking for more independent living. Youth hostels and some religious-based institutes can offer inexpensive alternatives to a hotel. If you have a car, you can opt to stay outside the city either in the nearby countryside in renovated farm buildings in an *agriturismo* or in a hotel above Florence in the hills near Fiesole or Piazzale Michelangelo. Hotels outside of the city will offer free parking, often swimming pools (although not always accessible to wheelchair users) and, especially in the torrid summer months, cooler air in the evenings. Whatever you decide to do, make sure to reserve well in advance, especially when coming between March and October. Remember that hotel prices are not written in stone, and depending on the season or other circumstances, many hotels may be willing to reduce their price especially if tourists are scarce. Even some very expensive hotels in the dead heat of the summer during July and August sometimes slash their prices since European tourists tend to abandon the cities to head for the beach or the mountains. Off-season prices are sometimes reduced by as much as 50 percent.

Notwithstanding Italian legislation, respect for laws concerning accessibility varies widely, and standards seem to be independent of the price you pay. Staying in a more expensive place is no guarantee of its accessibility. Remember no situation is going to be 100 percent perfect, and you may have to compromise on a hotel that may have generally good accessibility inside but an annoying step at the front door. If such be the case, the staff will usually be more than willing to help you over that difficulty. In conducting the surveys, one fairly consistent problem arose regarding the benches in roll-in showers. What is allowed by law is a mounted, fold-down seat, often quite small, usually unpadded and almost always without armrests. If this type of seat is unsuitable for you, then don't hesitate to ask that the hotel procure a safer one according to your requirements. Sometimes a simple plastic garden chair with armrests and four solid legs will be the easiest solution to the problem and will certainly be safer than dangerously perching on a tiny bench, but in a good hotel you should certainly insist on something far better. Indications are always made as to what type of seating is provided in the shower. The descriptions of the placement of grab bars which you will find below are always given as you face the WC or shower, unless otherwise indicated.

The APT (Azienda per il Turismo) publishes a yearly *Guide to Tourist Accommodation,* available both in city tourist information centers and on Internet: *www.firenzeturismo.it.* The home page has an English version, but the search engine is in Italian. Listings include all types of accommodations not only for the city of Florence but for the entire province of Florence as well, including Chianti, and range from hotels (*alberghi*) to B&B (*affittacamere*), residences and staying on a farm (*agriturismo*). The familiar international symbol of the wheelchair used to indicate accessibility (*accesso handicappati*), however, will not always indicate a truly accessible situation. It might list a hotel with an adapted room but will not alert you to the three high steps at the hotel entrance. Or an "accessible" entrance may be by means of a steep ramp through a back door leading to rooms whose bathrooms have no grab bars and a bathtub instead of a roll-in shower. Thus, be cautious if using this source and make sure to follow up any choices with a phone call asking specific questions.

The following entries contain detailed descriptions of accessibility and have been arranged according to price category; in general, and when applicable, based on the high season price of a double room.

Luxury (Above €400)

Hotel Savoy *****
Piazza della Repubblica, 7
50123 Florence
Tel: 055 27 351
Toll free: Italy 800-822-005
Toll free: USA 1-800-223-6800
Fax: 055 273 5888
E-mail: *reservations@hotelsavoy.it*
Home Page: *www.rfhotels.com*

Location: Within the pedestrian zone in the heart of the city's historic center.

General Description: This is a luxury hotel with 107 rooms; five doubles are accessible to wheelchair users. Contemporary-style rooms are equipped with air-conditioning, two-line phones, voice messaging, data port, fax, TV, minibar, safe. With conference room, bar, restaurant. Special menus are available on request.

Accessibility: Entrance with doorman is at street level. High reception desk. Public-accessible restroom in basement. Elevator door width: 105 centimeters (41 ¼ inches); cabin width: 175 centimeters (68 ⁷/₈ inches); cabin length: 140 centimeters (55 inches). Horizontal grab bar at rear of cabin; raised letter and Braille signage; audible car arrival signals.

General Description: A wheelchair-accessible room is located on each of the five floors. Three of these rooms can be connected to an adjoining room. Each room has lowered peephole on door, entrance hall, walk-in closet, two bathrooms: one adapted, one non-adapted, but accessible to wheelchair. Rooms have parquet flooring; double bed (58 centimeters [22 ¾ inches] high). Cramped maneuvering space without removing or rearranging furniture. High temperature control panel (temperature can also be controlled in individual rooms from the front desk). Adapted bathroom: roll-in shower with alarm, no grab bars, no shower seat; ergonomic sink with plastic tubing; WC with no grab bars.

Hotel Villa la Vedetta***
Viale Michelangelo, 78
50125 Florence
Tel: 055 681 631
Fax: 055 658 2544
E-mail: *info@villalavedetta.com*
Home Page: *www.hotelvillalavedetta.com*

Location: Near Piazzale Michelangelo on a hill overlooking Florence.

General Description: Situated in a lovely nineteenth-century villa just a stone's throw from Piazzale Michelangelo, this newly opened, five-star hotel has an equally spectacular view from its terrace overlooking Florence and the Arno. Eighteen rooms and suites offer individual air-conditioning and heating units, minibar, safe, telephone, satellite TV, computer with high-speed modem connection, radio, CD player, marble-paneled bathrooms with

Jacuzzi. The ample, traditionally landscaped grounds, with a swimming pool on the lower level, offer an interesting contrast to the slick, sophisticated modern interior decor. Full restaurant service, ample parking, and non-accessible shuttle service to town are available. Pets are welcome. About a ten-minute taxi ride to the center of town.

Accessibility: The two wheelchair-accessible (deluxe category) double rooms are located in an annex next to the villa. The entrance to each room is from the exterior through a small terrace set up with tables and chairs. There is a five-centimeter (2-inch) threshold lip. Doors open with key and have easy-grasp large handles.

Room No. 301 has double bed (57 centimeters [22 ½ inches] high) approachable from both sides, accessible desk, and wall closets with lower clothes rack for easy reach from wheelchair. There is marble flooring in both bedroom and bath. Spacious bath measures 375 by 175 centimeters (approximately 12 feet by 5 feet 9 inches) and has double sink with electronic eye faucet, low mirror; suspended bidet; suspended WC (55 centimeters [21 ⅝ inches] high) with retractable grab bar on left, transfer space on right; bathtub (59 centimeters [23 ¼ inches] high) has one fixed horizontal grab bar on back wall next to shower unit with flexible hose and lever-operated controls. There are also twist faucets for the tub. Portable tub bench can be provided on request.

Double Room No. 302 and bath are identical in typology to Room No. 301 with the exception of a roll-in shower instead of tub. Roll-in shower has a very slight incline towards the floor drain, both a fixed shower head and shower head on a flexible hose. There is a single lever-operated control for both shower units. Unpadded, fold-down small shower seat without armrests is 51 centimeters (20 inches) high. When seated, there is a diagonal grab bar on the wall to the left in a position which is slightly forward with respect to the bench, more useful to pull to stand than for transfer from a wheelchair.

The main floor of the villa has a luminous large double sitting room, dining room for breakfast and lunch, reception area, access to the panoramic terrace, and elevator to the lower level (cabin width: 100 centimeters [39 ³/8 inches]; cabin length: 120 centimeters [47 ¼ inches]). From the elevator, you exit to the main dining room and to the lower gardens. The outdoor Jacuzzi pool can be reached by wheelchair, but there are two steps down to the level of the swimming pool area.

Comments: Except for the threshold lip, entrance to the room is easily accessible, and the bathroom is, without a doubt, the largest accessible bath you will find in Florence. The annex is just a few meters from the entrance to the villa along an accessible paved route.

Expensive (€250-€400)

Hotel Bernini Palace**
Piazza San Firenze, 29
50122 Florence
Tel: 055 288 621
Fax: 055 268 272
E-mail: *bernini.firenze@baglionihotels.com*
Home Page: *www.baglionihotels.com*

Location: Central, just behind the Palazzo Vecchio and Piazza della Signoria.

General Description: This eighty-five-room hotel has been operating since the nineteenth century when, known as *Lo Scudo di Francia*, it served as residence for members of Parliament during the brief period when Florence was capital of the Kingdom of Italy. There are three wheelchair-accessible rooms: one on the 4° *piano* (fifth floor); two on the 2° *piano* (third floor). All rooms are equipped with air-conditioning, satellite color TV, telephone, hairdryer, minibar. Pets are welcome. Breakfast is served in the elegant *Sala del Parlamento* on the 1° *piano* (second floor).

Accessibility: The main entrance has a revolving door. A secondary wheelchair-accessible entrance (with threshold lip: 6 centimeters

[2 ³/₈ inches]) is just down the street at Borgo de' Greci, 27. Since this door is normally kept locked, the staff must be alerted to open the door. There is a narrow sidewalk in front of both doors (width: 43 centimeters [17 inches] with a 5-centimeter [2-inch] curb). The high doorbell to the right of the main entrance cannot be reached from a wheelchair. Main lobby has high reception desk, low-pile, wall-to-wall carpeting, no accessible restroom on ground floor, two steps up to bar area with a few tables set up for bar service in the lobby. Elevator has raised and Braille signage, audible signals, and measures 109 centimeters (just under 43 inches) wide, 168 centimeters (66 ¹/₈ inches) deep. The two doors on the short ends of the elevator are each 69 centimeters (27 ¼ inches) wide.

Wheelchair-accessible Room No. 401 (4° *piano*/fifth floor) is a two-bedroom suite with three bathrooms. The adapted bathroom is located off the small-entry hallway next to the accessible bedroom. Second bedroom with double bed (not separable) is upstairs. (If only the downstairs bedroom is needed, the upstairs bedroom will not be rented to someone else.) Downstairs bedroom has box spring double bed (can be separated): 63 centimeters (24 ¾ inches) high. Space on left side of bed (nearest door) is 112 centimeters (44 inches), telephone on bedside table, low-pile carpeting. Window facing east onto quiet courtyard; window closure: 147 centimeters (58 inches) high. Clearance between foot of bed and door to second bathroom: 67 centimeters (26 ³/₈ inches). (Note: This bathroom is not adapted and has a tub.) Adapted bathroom: Door (87 centimeters [34 ¼ inches]) swings out. Measurements of bathroom are 160 centimeters by 210 centimeters (approximately 5 feet 3 inches by just under 7 feet). WC has incorporated bidet with bidet control on right wall; retractable grab bar on left (no grab bar on right). Height of WC is 55 centimeters (just 19 ¾ inches) with easy-push flush mechanism on wall behind. Ergonomic sink has regulated height, wrapped pipe, tilted mirror, lever-operated faucet. Shower, measuring 80 by 80 centimeters (31 ½ by 31 ½ inches), has a plastic bottom with no-skid rubber mat and is slightly lowered with respect to the floor level in the rest of the bathroom. With alarm, horizontal grab bars on two walls, twist faucet controls.

Flexible hose can be hand held; shower head can be raised and lowered; no shower seat.

Wheelchair-accessible Room No. 201 faces street and has a small living room. Space on left side of double bed (side nearest bathroom) is 80 centimeters (31 ½ inches). Dimensions of bathroom: 250 by 170 centimeters (approximately 8 by 5 ½ feet). Door to bathroom opens inward. Retractable grab bar to left of WC, bidet control on right wall but no grab bar. Sink and shower characteristics as described above.

Wheelchair-accessible Room No. 202 is a large room with windows facing north onto Piazza San Firenze. Dimensions of bathroom are 160 by 200 centimeters (approximately 5 ¼ by 6 ½ feet). Door swings out. WC has incorporated bidet with bidet control on left wall, single retractable grab bar to right. Sink and shower characteristics as described above.

Comments: If you can afford it, Room No. 202 is the most spacious. Because the shower area in all three bathrooms is slightly lower with respect to the level of the bathroom floor, there is no level transfer space either into the shower or to the side of the WC. Therefore, these bathrooms may be more suitable for people who can manage a few steps. Although there is no shower bench, a hotel with these prices can easily acquire one if you ask. Also to consider is the revolving door at the entrance with the high doorbell and the necessity of going down the street to the secondary locked entrance without a doorbell.

Hotel Carolus**
Via XVII Aprile, 3
50129 Florence
Tel: 055 264 5539
Fax: 055 264 5550
E-mail: *info@carolushotel.com*
Home Page: *www.carolushotel.com*

Location: Between Piazza Indipendenza and Piazza San Marco.

General Description: Attractive newer hotel (opened September 2001) with fifty-three rooms. Four double and one single accessible rooms. Breakfast room, bar, sitting rooms, and accessible restroom on ground floor. All rooms with minibar, TV, and air-conditioning.

Accessibility: Automatic sliding doors at entrance. Entrance is level with street. High reception desk. Elevator to upper floors (door width: 80 centimeters [31 ½ inches]; cabin width: 94 centimeters [37 inches]; cabin length: 129 centimeters [50 ¾ inches]). With raised signage and audible car arrival signal. Wheelchair-accessible restroom on ground floor near bar (with grab bar to right, transfer space to left of WC). Breakfast room tables have central pedestal legs but allow adequate depth for seating with wheelchair. Public spaces have wall-to-wall, low-pile carpeting. Rooms have wooden parquet floors.

Rooms No. 111 and No. 311 are quiet, spacious back rooms with double bed. Wheelchair access from both sides of bed. Bed can be separated.

Room No. 212 double. Cramped spaces in room and narrow entrance create difficulty for wheelchair users especially in opening door to bathroom.

Room No. 103 single. Small room on street with similar narrow entrance creating some extra maneuvering in opening bathroom door if using a wheelchair. Removing desk at the foot of bed would create extra space in this small room.

Bathrooms. (180 by 210 centimeters [6 by 7 feet]) have tile floors, roll-in showers with horizontal grab bar on one wall, shower spray unit with hose and soap dish at 150 centimeters (59 inches) from floor, shower chair with back but no arms can be provided on request by the hotel. Ergonomic sink has low mirror, lever-operated faucet, plastic-wrapped pipe. WC (52 centimeters [21 ½ inches] high) with easy-flush panel, horizontal grab bar on right wall too distant (approximately 5 centimeters [2 inches] from front of and not next to toilet). Handheld bidet shower spray unit to left of WC.

Comments: This bright, attractive hotel, decorated in tones of yellow and red, has a good location and, rare for Florence, an easily accessible entrance.

Hotel degli Orafi**
Lungarno Archibusieri, 4
50121 Firenze
Tel: 055 26 622
Fax: 055 266 2111
Home Page: *www.hoteldegliorafi.com*

Location: On the Arno between Ponte Vecchio and the Uffizi.

General Description: This medium-size hotel with forty-two rooms opened in 2002 and occupies part of a former *pensione* that provided the panoramic vista for the film *Room with a View*. While many of the rooms look out on the river, the four wheelchair-accessible rooms face quiet courtyards, some with a special cropped detail of the Duomo. Many of the public rooms have original frescoes and are tastefully and comfortably decorated, giving the impression of being in an elegant home.

Accessibility: The wide entrance is level with the street and has an automatic door. With high reception desk. Elevator to upper floors, with raised and Braille signage and audible signals, has two doors at right angles. Elevator door width: 78 centimeters (30 ¾ inches); cabin width and length each 120 centimeters (47 ¼ inches). Upstairs public rooms (bar, library, sitting room, breakfast room) are all accessible with a platform lift to the main part of the breakfast room. Two steps (no ramp) to the terrace off the bar on the top floor.

Room Nos. 404, 304, 205, 103 are wheelchair accessible. Tastefully furnished rooms have parquet floors, open-frame double bed (can be separated and measures 63 ½ centimeters [25 inches] high), clear pathways, telephone on table next to bed, TV with remote control, minibar. Light switches and thermostat controls are reachable from a wheelchair; window closure is 148 centimeters

(58 ¼ inches) high. High clothes rod in closet. All **bathrooms** are large and have corner roll-in showers (80 by 80 centimeters [31 ½ by 31 ½ inches]) with swinging glass doors (both can be opened), grab bars on two walls (for Nos. 304 and 404 only), alarm, lever faucet, flexible hose (also hand held), no shower seat. Standard high-back WC (43 centimeters [17 inches] high) has button-flush mechanism, fixed horizontal grab bar (on left wall for Room No. 304; on right wall for Room No. 404). Encased sink (82 centimeters [32 ¼ inches] high with knee clearance of 75 centimeters [29 ½ inches]) has lever-operated faucet, unwrapped metal pipe, low mirror. Bidet (low, no grab bars).

Comments: The level of accessibility in this hotel is among the best in Florence. Room No. 304 is more suitable than No. 404 for larger wheelchairs, because the door to the room can be opened slightly wider. Room No. 205 and No. 103 have no grab bars in the bathroom.

Hotel Kraft** **
Via Solferino, 2
50123 Florence
Tel: 055 284 273
Fax: 055 239 8267
E-mail: *info@krafthotel.it*
Home Page: *www.krafthotel.it*

Location: In a quiet residential area west of the historic center across the street from the Teatro Comunale, two blocks from the Arno.

General Description: This comfortable, old-style, eighty-room hotel has a rooftop terrace, with a swimming pool, offering panoramic views of the city and the surrounding hills. Presently there is one wheelchair-accessible double; a newly renovated second wheelchair-accessible double will be available by June 2004. Future plans include renovation of the fifth floor with several additional accessible rooms. Rooms and public spaces have traditional decor. Amenities include minibar, color satellite and pay TV, direct-dial telephone, air-conditioning. Full restaurant service is offered with buffet breakfast served on the roof garden during the late spring and summer months.

Accessibility: Wheelchair-accessible entrance is presently through a secondary door in Via Montebello, 29/A. The main entrance will become wheelchair-accessible with the installation of a stair lift in the lobby planned for autumn 2004. There is an adapted but very small WC on the ground floor (no lateral transfer space with clearance space in front of the WC measuring 94 centimeters [37 inches] wide by 98 centimeters [38 ⅝ inches] deep). Two elevators to upper floors (cabin depth is presently 120 centimeters [47 ¼ inches]) will also be renovated by mid 2004. Small **double Room No. 125** has entrance foyer and bedroom with parquet floors. Double bed (56 centimeters [22 inches] high). There is a very narrow space on each side of the bed, and in order to approach the bed from a wheelchair, the bed will have to be pushed to the wall, creating a maximum space of 83 centimeters (32 ⅝ inches) to one side of the bed. There is room at the foot of the bed, between the bed and desk and the window for maneuvering with an average-size manual wheelchair. The spacious bathroom with marble floor and paneling measures 270 by 160 centimeters (approximately 8 feet 10 inches by 5 feet 3 inches) and has a roll-in shower with lever-operated faucet and flexible hose that can be hand held, alarm; no shower seat. WC (53 centimeters [21 inches] high), in proximity to the shower, has handheld shower bidet and retractable grab bar on left; room for left transfer, push-button flush mechanism on right wall. The sink can be raised or lowered and has a lever-operated faucet, lowered mirror, and insulated pipe; hair dryer, light sockets, shelves on right wall are placed for easy reach from a wheelchair. Two narrow track ramps (each 24 centimeters [9 ½ inches] wide) are placed over the one step between the elevator and corridor to reach this room. The large, wheelchair-accessible double with adapted bathroom (tub and roll-in shower) which will be ready by June 2004 is connected to an adjoining double with non-adapted bathroom. The rooftop terrace with swimming pool is wheelchair-accessible.

Comments: The architect who designed the bathroom in Room No. 125 has paid particular attention to important design details in rendering maximum accessibility. Continuing in this vein, plans to modify the lobby entrance and elevator, together with the addition of the new double on the fourth floor and future plans to build several wheelchair-accessible rooms on the fifth floor, will give this hotel additional accessibility. A shower chair can be furnished on request.

Hotel Pierre****
Via Lamberti, 5
50123 Firenze
Tel: 055 216 218
Fax: 055 239 6573
E-mail: *pierre@remarhotels.com*
Home Page: *www.remarhotels.com*

Location: Near the main post office and Piazza della Repubblica.

General Description: A very centrally located, forty-four-room hotel. Rooms have air-conditioning, telephone, TV, minibar. Buffet breakfast served in ground-floor breakfast room. Two accessible doubles and two singles with semi-adapted bathrooms. Plans are underway to add two new rooms with fully adapted bathrooms in 2004.

Accessibility: Main entrance is through a revolving door with side doors to the immediate left and right. One step (11 centimeters [4 3/8 inches]) at the right side door which is normally kept locked but is easily visible from the reception desk. Ground-floor rooms are level with exception of one step to bar area. Elevator (door width: 80 centimeters [31 ½ inches]) measures 109 centimeters (3 feet 7 inches) square. Raised signage, no Braille. Rooms inspected: include spacious **doubles No. 503 and No. 501** with parquet floor, open-frame large double bed (beds can be separated) 55 centimeters (21 5/8 inches) high. Bathroom (Room No. 503) has roll-in shower with accordion-like doors that pull to close; lever-operated faucet; flexible hose can be hand held. No shower seat, no grab bars. Sink with wrapped pipe and twist faucets. WC is suspended, 54 centimeters (21 ½ inches) high, with easy-push mechanism on back wall, no grab bars. Bidet. **Singles No. 502 and No. 508** have ample space in room. Their large bathrooms have similar typology to that of No. 503.

Comments: Semi-adapted bathrooms are without grab bars and shower seat. Rooms are spacious. Doors are opened with normal keys. Runner carpet in upstairs hall outside of elevator.

Hotel Villa Gabriele d'Annunzio**
Via Gabriele d'Annunzio 141 a-b
50135 Florence
Tel: 055 602 960
Fax: 055 619 3113
E-mail: *hotel.dannunzio@tin.it*
Home Page: *www.hotel-dannunzio.com*

Location: In a residential area below the hill town of Settignano, about fifteen minutes by car from the center of Florence.

General Description: An eighty-room hotel located in a restored ex-monastery surrounded by gardens, ample parking, small swimming pool. Grounds and hotel are decorated with contemporary sculpture. No restaurant. Breakfast room. All rooms have minibar, TV, air-conditioning, sound proofing, Internet connection. Two conference rooms in basement. Larger room holds 140 people.

Accessibility: One step to porch with small ramp located at left end of porch near designated parking spaces.

Four wheelchair-accessible Rooms No. 11 (ground floor), and Nos. 117, 217, 318. All have spacious bathrooms with terracotta floors. Showers have sunken base but are fitted with an aluminum panel to become flush with floor. Shower benches are fitted onto L-shaped grab bar on shower wall, alarm in shower. Low mirror over ergonomic sink. Bidet. WC has no grab bars. Room Nos. 11 and 318 are larger with wheelchair access from both sides of bed. Room No. 217 can connect to adjoining No. 218 (with non-adapted bathroom). Two elevators to all floors. Dimensions of door are 80 centimeters (31 ½ inches); cabin width: 110 centimeters (43 ¼ inches); cabin length: 140 centimeters (55 ⅛ inches). Raised signage, audible signals. Adapted bathroom on ground floor next to breakfast room.

Comments: This rather anonymous hotel caters largely to business meetings and tour groups (Grand Circle). Heavy iron furniture in breakfast room. Questionable stability of aluminum floor panel in roll-in showers. Room Nos. 117 and 217 are small. Spaces between the cement blocks of walk to swimming pool make unassisted transit in wheelchair impossible.

Moderate (€100-€200)

Convitto della Calza
Piazza della Calza, 6
50125 Florence
Tel: 055 222 287
Fax: 055 223 912
E-mail: *calza@calza.it*
Home Page: *http://www.calza.it*

Location: Just inside the city gate of Porta Romana on the south side of Florence. About four miles from the "Certosa" exit of the A1 Autostrada and the Superstrada Firenze-Siena.

Transportation: Wheelchair-accessible city Bus Nos. 12 and 13 stop in Piazzale Porta Romana just outside the gate; Wheelchair-accessible Bus No. 11 stops in Piazza Calza opposite the Convitto. Taxi stand in Piazzale Porta Romana. Parking available just inside the city gate in the parking lot next to the Convitto. Two designated spaces near the entrance on the left for disability parking permit holders.

General Description: Located in a former convent founded in the fourteenth century, the recently restored Convitto, administrated by the Curia, now functions as a conference center and hotel. Ten single, twenty double, and six triple rooms (some simply furnished in keeping with the spirit of the convent, others furnished with antiques) are equipped with private bath, telephone, television, air-conditioning, and Internet connection. There are four wheelchair-accessible rooms. Breakfast (included in room price) is served from 7:30-9:30 in the dining room on the 1° *piano*/second floor. Lunch and dinner (half— and full-board pension plan) available. The seating capacity of the six conference rooms ranges from twenty to four hundred. Adjacent parking lot offers 20 percent discount rate to guests of the Convitto; designated parking spaces are free with appropriate permit.

Accessibility: Ramp at entrance through automatic glass doors. High reception desk. Short, low metal ramps at door to courtyard and in loggia area to overcome slight level changes. Dimensions of elevator to rooms are door width: 75 centimeters (29 ½ inches); cabin width: 78 centimeters (30 ¾ inches); cabin depth: 124 centimeters (48 ¾ inches). Raised number and Braille signage. Audible signals. Elevator to breakfast room on 1° *piano* (second floor) has same dimensions and characteristics. Elevator to basement auditorium and public restrooms with door width: 85 centimeters (33 ½ inches); cabin width: 135 centimeters (53 ⅛ inches); cabin length: 145 centimeters (57 ⅛ inches). Public men's and women's restrooms on basement level with retractable grab bar next to WC and ergonomic sink which can be raised and lowered. Four wheelchair-accessible double rooms have adapted or partially adapted bathrooms. All doors have knob mechanism and open with keys. Two accessible rooms on the 1° *piano* (second floor) overlooking the courtyard are:

Room No. 113 double with double bed (57 centimeters [22 ½ inches] high). Space to right of bed: 78 centimeters (30 ¾ inches) to left of bed space narrows to 57 centimeters (22 ½ inches) due to presence of chest of drawers, then widens to 123 centimeters (48 ⅜ inches) next to head of bed. Partially adapted bathroom has tile floor; enclosed box shower (height of shower base: 4 centimeters [1 ⅝ inches]); shower doors open out. Ergonomic sink has insulated pipe, mirror with adjustable inclination. WC has horizontal and vertical grab bars on left; retractable grab bar on right.

Room No. 114. Double with twin beds. With present arrangement space between beds measures 75 centimeters (29 ½ inches), with 110 centimeters (43 ¼ inches) between right bed and wall. Partially adapted bathroom with tile floor (measures 180 by 205 centimeters [5 ¾ by 6 ¾ feet]) has roll-in shower, alarm cord, horizontal grab bar on left wall only, no shower seat. Ergonomic sink with lever-operated faucet, insulated pipe, tilted mirror. WC has handheld shower bidet, easy-push flush panel, grab bar on right wall somewhat distant from WC.

Two accessible rooms on the 2° *piano* (third floor) overlooking the courtyard:

Room No. 20. Double with twin beds. Room is quite small. Beds: 60 centimeters (23 ⁵/₈ inches) high. Space between beds: 78 centimeters (30 ¾ inches). Space between foot of bed and wall: 82 centimeters (32 ¼ inches). Space between left bed and wardrobe (in front of door to bathroom) 55 centimeters (21 ⁵/₈ inches). Height of window-opening device: 142 centimeters (just under 56 inches). Fully adapted bathroom (measures 280 by 180 centimeters [9 by 6 feet]), has tile floor, corner roll-in shower with mounted, fold-down shower bench, alarm cord, lever-operated faucet. WC (52 centimeters [20 ½ inches] high) with retractable grab bar on left; horizontal and vertical grab bars on right wall. Ergonomic sink with insulated pipe; mirror with adjustable inclination.

Room No. 221. Double with twin beds. Door to bathroom easily accessible. Possibility of rearranging beds. Distance between beds with present arrangement: 110 centimeters (3 feet 7 ³/₈ inches). Fully adapted bathroom (measures 285 by 175 centimeters [9 ¼ by 5 ¾ feet]), has tile floor; corner roll-in shower with alarm on cord, horizontal grab bars on both walls, mounted fold-down shower bench, lever-operated faucet. WC with alarm and horizontal grab bar on right wall, retractable grab bar on left, standard metal push flush device on left wall. Ergonomic sink with insulated pipe. Inclination of mirror can be adjusted.

Comments: For convenience of parking, tranquility, cleanliness, and price, the Convitto offers one of the better possibilities in Florence for accessible lodging. Good wheelchair accessibility in public spaces. Decor is simple but tasteful. Green lawns are in the middle of the large central courtyard; public seating areas are arranged under its surrounding loggia. With the exception of no room service and no public bar or minibar in the rooms, the Convitto easily ranks with an upgrade three-star hotel.

Grand Hotel Mediterraneo*
Lungarno del Tempio, 44
50121 Florence
Tel: 055 660 241
Fax: 055 679 560
E-mail: *info@hotelmediterraneo.com*
Home Page: *www.hotelmediterraneo.com*

Location: On the north bank of the Arno near the San Niccolò bridge, about 1.5 kilometers ($^9/_{10}$ mile) from the Ponte Vecchio. Wheelchair-accessible Bus D stops in Piazza Ferrucci on the opposite side of the river. Easily reached from the "Firenze-Sud" exit of the A1 autostrada. Parking available.

General Description: A very large (331 rooms) modern hotel with three restaurants (only one is wheelchair accessible), bar, conference rooms. Pets welcome except in dining rooms. Rooms are equipped with telephone, air-conditioning, color TV, hair dryer.

Accessibility: Six steps at entrance with platform lift for wheelchair users. No call button (hotel personnel must be alerted to operate lift). Automatic doors. Large public spaces. High counters at reception desk and bar. Restaurant in main lobby is wheelchair accessible. Possibility of special dietary menu with advance notice. One wheelchair-accessible restroom on ground floor (in men's room).

Elevator—door width: 76 centimeters (slightly under 30 inches); cabin width: 124 centimeters (48 ¾ inches); cabin depth: 95 centimeters (37 ³/₈ inches). **Eight wheelchair-accessible rooms:** six triple rooms with one double and one single bed; two double rooms with double bed only. Doors to rooms: stationary knob on outside, push to open after swiping key, lever handle inside. No lowered rack in closets. Windows have pull curtains and raised blinds, mechanism to raise and lower blinds within reach of person in wheelchair. The triples are more spacious than the smaller doubles. Bathrooms in all accessible rooms have tile floors, roll-in showers with horizontal grab bars, handheld shower head, four plastic shower chairs available on request. Ergonomic sink with plastic pipe, high non-tilted mirror. WC has retractable grab bar with handheld bidet shower unit.

Hotel Benivieni*
Via delle Oche, 5
50122 Firenze
Tel: 055 238 2133
Fax: 055 239 8248
E-mail: *info@hotelbenivieni.it*
Home Page: *www.hotelbenivieni.it*

Location: Between the Duomo and Piazza della Repubblica.

General Description: A small (fifteen rooms) hotel located in the heart of the *centro storico* with two wheelchair-accessible rooms. Soundproof, air-conditioned rooms have satellite TV, telephone, safe. Garage facilities and Internet connection are available. Buffet breakfast is included in price of room.

Accessibility: Main entrance is through heavy wrought-iron double glass doors: one step (10 centimeters [4 inches]) from a narrow sidewalk (72 centimeters [28 ³/₈ inches]wide) with a 10-centimeter (4-inch) curb. The ramped, wheelchair-accessible entrance to the right is normally kept locked but is easily visible from the reception desk. Elevator with automatic door, width: 78 centimeters (30 ¾ inches); cabin width: 82 centimeters (32 ¼ inches); cabin length: 120 centimeters (47 ¼ inches). **Spacious double No. 201** with key card to open, parquet floor, double open-frame bed (beds can be separated) 52 centimeters (20 ½ inches) high, has bath with roll-in shower. Bathroom measures 220 centimeters by 165 centimeters (approximately 7 feet 2 inches by 4 feet 5 inches). WC has retractable grab bar on left, no grab bar on right wall, easy-push button flush, handheld bidet shower unit on right wall. Corner roll-in shower has alarm, lever-operated faucet, flexible hose that can be hand held, horizontal grab bars on two walls, glass doors which have a maximum opening of 76 centimeters (30 inches). Hotel can provide a four-legged chair without armrests for the shower. Sink has wrapped pipe, lever-operated faucet, low mirror. **Single No. 90** on ground floor. Ramp to door. Ample room has parquet floor, "French" bed (narrow double bed). Bath is of same size and characteristics as bathroom described above with the exception that the shower is open (without doors). There is a second non-adapted bathroom in this room.

Comments: Great location. The sidewalk curb creates the necessity of assistance at entrance to this hotel. Ground floor is barrier free with ramp to breakfast room. The narrow opening of the shower in Room No. 201 may be a problem for transfer into the shower from a wheelchair. The bathroom door of Room No. 90 opens out into the entrance foyer of the room, narrowing passage into the room to 74 centimeters (just over 29 inches) leaving little space to maneuver for larger power chairs or scooters. A normal four-legged unpadded metal chair without armrests is provided for use in the shower.

Hotel Botticelli***
Via Taddea, 8
50123 Firenze
Tel: 055 290 905

Fax: 055 294 322
E-mail: *botticelli@italyhotel.com*
Home Page: *www.venere.it/firenze/botticelli*

Location: Near the San Lorenzo Market.

General Description: A small, thirty-four room hotel with two (double and single) wheelchair-accessible rooms with partially adapted bathrooms, telephone, TV, air-conditioning. Serves buffet breakfast. Has a bar. Parking with hotel discount in nearby garage. Small upstairs terrace has partial views of the Duomo and Giotto's bell tower.

Accessibility: Two steps at entrance, narrow sidewalk, high doorbell to right of door. Wheelchair-accessible entrance is through the hotel garage to the immediate left of the main entrance. Elevator from garage level to all floors. Elevator dimensions are door and cabin width: 81 centimeters (31 $^7/_8$ inches); cabin depth: 173 centimeters (68 $^1/_8$ inches). Raised letter and Braille signage. Audible arrival signal. Breakfast room tables have a central pedestal making it difficult for wheelchair to fit under table. High counter at bar. Accessible public restroom in basement.

Double No. 108 (1° *piano*/second floor). Double bed is accessible from left side only. Low pile wall-to-wall carpet. Maneuvering space immediately to left between door to room and bed and immediately to right between bedroom door and bathroom. Tight maneuvering space in rest of bedroom. Bathroom (283 by 172 centimeters [approximately 9 by 5 feet]) has tile floor. Roll-in shower with lever-operated controls, alarm on cord, no shower seat, horizontal grab bars on both walls in shower area. Ergonomic sink has wrapped pipe and lever-operated faucet, low mirror, hair dryer. WC has easy panel-flush mechanism, no grab bars.

Note: This is a quiet room overlooking a small internal light well, no view. Request that the telephone be put on the table on the left side of the bed.

Single Room No. 116 (1° *piano*/second floor). Single bed with desk and small wardrobe, low pile wall-to-wall carpet. Good maneuvering space. Window on internal light well, no view. Bathroom (265 by 192 centimeters [approximately 8 feet 6 inches by 6 feet 5 inches]) has tile floor. Roll-in shower with horizontal grab bars on both walls, alarm, no shower seat, lever-operated controls. Ergonomic sink has lever-operated controls, low mirror, hair dryer. WC, easy-flush mechanism, horizontal grab bar on right side only (shared with shower).

Comments: If you can overlook the inconvenience of entering through the garage, this small hotel is quiet, tasteful, but unpretentious and is located in one of the most characteristic neighborhoods of the historic center. The staff is extremely friendly and willing to help. Although the front doorbell is too high to reach from the seated position of a wheelchair, the reception desk is immediately opposite the glass front door. A staff member will open garage door for wheelchair access. Hotel garage has a few parking spaces, and you need to make a special request if you want to park your car there. Otherwise, the nearby garage has valet service.

Hotel de la Pace***
Via La Marmora, 28
50121 Firenze
Tel: 055 577 343
Fax: 055 577 576
E-mail: *info@hoteldelapace.it*
Home Page: *www.hoteldelapace.it*

Location: One block from Viale Matteotti, three blocks from Piazza San Marco. About fifteen minutes from Piazza del Duomo.

General Description: An attractive medium-sized (forty-two rooms) hotel with one wheelchair-accessible room. Ground-floor public rooms recently redecorated. Lounge, breakfast room, bar, and accessible restroom on ground floor. Buffet breakfast served. Rooms equipped with TV, air-conditioning, telephone, minibar, and hairdryer.

Accessibility: Ramp at entrance. Manual double swinging glass doors. High reception desk. Accessible restroom on ground floor. Restroom measures 165 by 209 centimeters (approximately 5 ½ by 7 feet). Retractable grab bar on right side of WC; horizontal grab bar and hand shower unit on left (wall) side. Sink with lever faucet. **Small elevator:** door width: 60 centimeters (23 ⅝ inches); cabin width: 72 centimeters (28 ⅜ inches); cabin length: 113 centimeters (44 ½ inches).

Double Room No. 102 (second floor/1° *piano*) overlooks internal courtyard. Heavy entrance door opens with lever handle. High peephole. Entrance foyer to room: 144 by 114 centimeters (approximately 4 ¾ by 3 ¾ feet). Double bed can be separated. Adequate but not roomy space for maneuvering. Old-fashioned window with outside shutters with high closure will require assistance in opening and shutting. Bathroom: spacious, with glass door opening onto small balcony. Horizontal grab bar on wall to right of WC; alarm on cord to left. WC on raised platform (53 centimeters [20 ⅞ inches] high). Roll-in shower has vertical grab bar, mounted fold-down shower seat. Bidet. Sink with lever faucet, unwrapped pipe.

Comments: Management is gracious and willing to assist. Small elevator will limit accessibility to many. Heavy door to room may require assistance in opening. Hotels plans to expand; new accessible rooms will be available.

Hotel Galileo*
Via Nazionale, 22a
50123 Firenze
Tel: 055 496 645
Fax: 055 496 447
E-mail: *hgalileo@dada.it*

Location: One block south of Piazza Indipendenza. Not far from the San Lorenzo market and the Santa Maria Novella railroad station.

General Description: A small, twenty-eight-room hotel with two wheelchair-accessible rooms: double and single with adapted bathrooms. Breakfast room, bar on ground floor. Rooms equipped with TV, air-conditioning, telephone, minibar, safe. Have had clients in manual and power wheelchairs.

Accessibility: Step at entrance (approximately 15 centimeters [6 inches]); small wooden ramp is put in place when needed. Front desk is directly opposite door. No accessible restroom on ground floor. Dimensions of elevator are door width: 67 centimeters (26 $^3/_8$ inches); cabin width: 80 centimeters (31 ½ inches); cabin length: 116 centimeters (45 $^5/_8$ inches). Raised letter and Braille signage. Doors to rooms are easily opened by passing key cards in front of opening mechanism and do not have to be swiped. Push door to open. Lever handle inside. Narrow upstairs corridors lead to rooms. Companion dogs accepted.

Double No. 134 (third floor/2° *piano*): sleeps up to four people. Double bed; two single beds. Very spacious, well lit, looks over quiet internal courtyard, large bathroom, retractable grab bar and alarm button on left (wall) side of WC (52 centimeters [20 ½ inches] high), hand bidet shower to right of WC (requires reach). Ergonomic sink with lever-operated faucet. Shower has raised track (5 centimeters [2 inches]) for sliding doors (width of opening: 55 centimeters [21 $^5/_8$ inches]), mounted fold-down shower bench. No grab bars in shower but curved arms on bench offer some support. Alarm on cord in shower. Because the raised border and narrow opening do not permit transfer directly from a wheelchair, this situation is recommended for someone who can walk a few steps.

Single No. 124 (second floor/1° *piano*) with "French" (small double) bed looking over internal courtyard. Crowded furniture arrangement. Recommended for someone who can walk a few steps and who doesn't want much distance between furniture, or with some furniture rearrangement, for someone in a small manual wheelchair. The spacious bathroom is similar to the one described above in terms of size, sink, and shower with these exceptions: the retractable grab bar is on the right side of WC, alarm button on the left, hand shower next to toilet is within reach.

Hotel il Guelfo Bianco***
Via Cavour, 29
50129 Florence
Tel: 055 288 330-1
Fax: 055 295 203
E-mail: *info@ilguelfobianco.it*
Home Page: *www.ilguelfobianco.it*

Location: Central between Piazza del Duomo and Piazza San Marco.

General Description: This is a small, twenty-nine-room hotel with two wheelchair-accessible rooms on the ground floor. Rooms are equipped with air-conditioning, satellite TV, radio, telephone, minibar, safe, hairdryer. Breakfast room with garden court, bar, small seating area are on ground floor.

Accessibility: Threshold lip (2.5 centimeters [1 inch]) at entrance. High reception desk. Two wheelchair-accessible rooms include one **double (No. 4)** with two single beds (49.5 centimeters [19 ½ inches] high). Wardrobe has possibility of pulling clothes bar down to wheelchair level. Safe and thermometer control (height 156 centimeters [61 ½ inches]). Window closure is too high to be reached from a wheelchair. Glass door opens onto small courtyard. **Single (No. 3).** This is a small room but with adequate space. High window closure cannot be reached from a wheelchair. Bathroom (No. 4) sink has plastic tubing, lever-operated faucet. Alarm. WC with incorporated bidet, horizontal grab bar on left wall. Roll-in shower with horizontal grab bar, no shower bench. Bathroom (No. 3): Similar to bathroom described above.

Comments: Rooms are sparsely but adequately furnished with adequate maneuvering space. Both rooms give out onto small courtyard space, which is also reached by a door from the lobby area (possible fire escape route). This hotel has also had guests with scooters who found the spaces, both public and private, adequate for maneuvering.

Hotel Orto de'Medici*
Via San Gallo, 30
50129 Florence
Tel: 055 483 427
Fax: 055 461 276
E-mail: *hotel@ortodeimedici.it*

Location: One block west of Piazza San Marco.

General Description: A small hotel (thirty-one rooms) located on a quiet street in a charming nineteenth-century palace bordering a garden which once belonged to the Medici. Two attractively furnished, wheelchair-accessible double rooms are located on the *primo piano* (second floor) near the sitting and breakfast rooms. Rooms have air-conditioning, hair dryer, telephone, satellite TV, minibar. Internet access is available. Landscape frescoes decorate the walls of the breakfast room off of which is a terrace where evening drinks are served in summer months (one step 8 centimeters [3 1/8 inches] to terrace level). Overall atmosphere is that of a private, graceful home.

Accessibility: Double glass doors at entrance open inwards. High reception desk. Elevator to upper floors has raised and Braille signage (door width: 77 centimeters [30 1/4 inches]; cabin length: 122 centimeters [48 inches]).

Room No. 14 overlooking garden has over 100 centimeters (39 ½ inches) clearance to each side of bed; 95 centimeters (37 ½ inches) between foot of bed and wardrobe. Open-frame bed (can be separated) is 53 centimeters (just under 21 inches) high. High clothes rod in wardrobe. Air-conditioning control is reachable from wheelchair. Bathroom has roll-in shower with lever faucet control, flexible hose, alarm, no grab bars, sturdy shower chair available; WC is 48 centimeters (19 inches) high with easy, push-button flush, no grab bars, handheld bidet shower unit on flexible hose. Sink has lever faucet control, unwrapped pipes, and hair dryer. Door to bathroom is 73 centimeters (28 ¾ inches) wide, swings in; slight threshold lip.

Room No.15 has double bed (can be separated), tile floor, telephone next to bed, window closure 150 centimeters (59 inches). Bathroom has roll-in shower, WC, sink with same features as above.

Comments: There are presently no grab bars in the shower but a very sturdy shower chair with a back (but no arms) is available on request: 44 centimeters (17 ¼ inches) high with a 43-by-43-centimeter (17-square-inch) seat. Room No. 14's bathroom is larger. Management says grab bars are on order. In addition to its charm and good location, this hotel has overall good accessibility.

Hotel Porta Rossa*
Via Porta Rossa, 19
50123 Florence
Tel: 055 287 551
Fax: 055 282 179

Location: Central just off Via Tornabuoni and near the Strozzi Palace.

General Description: First opened as an inn in the fourteenth century, numerous luminaries have been guests at the Hotel Porta Rossa: Lord Byron, Stendahl, and Balzac, to name a few. Seventy-eight rooms; four are wheelchair accessible: two on the 1° *piano* (second floor); two on the 2° *piano* (third floor). All rooms are equipped with air-conditioning, satellite color TV, telephone, and hairdryer. Pets welcome. Public rooms on ground floor include billiard room, bar, breakfast room, TV room. Marble and parquet floors throughout. Wheelchair-accessible restroom on ground floor.

Accessibility: Entrance is from a narrow sidewalk—width: 77 centimeters (30 ¼ inches); curb: 9 centimeters (3 ½ inches). One step (20 centimeters [8 inches]). Encased doormat at entrance. Heavy double glass doors open out (each 69 centimeters [27 ¼ inches] wide). There is a wooden ramp available, placed when needed, and a doorbell outside the entrance on the right, reachable from sidewalk level. High reception desk in lobby. A wheelchair-accessible restroom is located on the ground floor. Elevator (88 centimeters [34 ⅝ inches] deep; 142 centimeters [56 inches] wide) with two doors (each 63 centimeters [24 ¾ inches] wide) placed at right angles. You enter on the long side and exit to the right on the short side. The elevator has no Braille, raised numbers, or audible signals. **Wheelchair-accessible Room No. 59** on the 2° *piano* (third floor) was inspected. This is a large room with parquet flooring; three single beds have open wooden frames; height of mattress of two beds: 54 centimeters (21 ¼ inches); third bed: 59 centimeters (23 ¼ inches). Telephone and lamp on table next to bed nearest bathroom. Bedroom window faces SW onto quiet side street. High window closure: 150 centimeters (59 inches). Large bathroom with tile floor (180 by 410 centimeters [approximately 6 by 14.5 feet]); WC (53 centimeters [just under 21 inches] high) with incorporated bidet faces door, retractable grab bar on left, horizontal and vertical grab bars on right wall. Easy-push flush and bidet with lever-controlled faucet on right wall. Ergonomic sink can be adjusted in height, has wrapped pipe, tilted mirror, and lever-operated faucet. Shower has raised edge and plastic bottom with concentric raised ridges for non-skid. Lower and right edge of shower base can be removed for "roll-in," although a slight rounded raised ridge still remains at the shower threshold. Mounted fold-down shower seat without arms and padding (50 centimeters [just under 19 ¾ inches] high). When seated, grab bar is on your left together with lever-operated shower controls (approximately 122 centimeters [48 inches] high) and alarm. The flexible hose (63 centimeters [just under 25 inches] long) can also be hand held. There is also a bathtub and a low-positioned house phone near the shower.

Comments: The Porta Rossa has a lot of character and Old World charm, albeit slightly dog eared. The wooden ramp must be positioned every time you leave or enter the hotel. Maneuvering in and out of the elevator and dealing with a shower that is not a true roll-in may present problems for some users.

Ingrid Affittacamere
Piazza San Salvi, 13
50135 Florence
Tel./Fax: 055 667 646
E-mail: *Ingrid.florence.rooms@tin.it*
Home Page: *www.ingridaffittacamere.it*

Location: In a typical residential neighborhood on the outskirts of Florence about two miles east of the Ponte Vecchio.

General Description: A sunny, three-room, ground-floor, and attractively furnished apartment consisting of entrance hall, two bedrooms, two and a half baths (one wheelchair-accessible), a multi-use kitchen, dining, living room with sofa bed (sleeps two), and a private terrace. Can sleep up to six people. Services include weekly linens, TV, heating, air conditioning.

Accessibility: There is a wooden ramp (120 centimeters [47 ¼"] wide) inside the main entrance door. Door to apartment is at the top of the ramp. Door widths within the apartment for the bedroom with accessible bath and for the accessible bath are 75 centimeters (29 ½"). Doors to the second bedroom and multi-use room measure 70 centimeters (27 ½"). The accessible bedroom has an open frame double bed (can be separated) with spaces to the left, right, and at the foot of the bed of 100 centimeters (39 ½") or slightly over. The accessible bathroom measures 140 by 200 centimeters (approximately 4 ½ by 6 ½ feet). Bathroom door opens inwards. WC, directly opposite the door, is 50 centimeters (19 ¾") high with a fixed grab bar on the right and retractable grab bar on the left. A handheld shower bidet unit is also on the left and within easy reach of the WC. The roll-in shower has a suspended unpadded shower seat with arm rests; no grab bars. The shower unit is on a flexible hose which can be hand held and there is a lever operated faucet on the wall on the right (when seated) and within close proximity of the shower seat. The ergonomic sink has a lever operated faucet and lowered mirror.

Comments: The inward opening door to the accessible bathroom somewhat cramps the space in front of the WC. Transfer to the shower seat is from the right side only (as if facing the seat) because of the proximity of the sink to the shower. Transportation will be needed to get to the center of town. Wheelchair-accessible Bus 20 passing through Piazza San Marco stops one block away. The owners live upstairs and Ingrid's husband is a cab driver for one of the companies which operate accessible taxis.

Palazzo Belfiore
Via dei Velluti, 8
50125 Florence
Tel: 055 61 115
Fax: 055 605 603
E-mail: *belfiore@dada.it*
Home Page: *www.residencebelfiore.it*

Location: Excellent location on a quiet side street in the Oltrarno just off Via Guicciardini between Palazzo Pitti and the Ponte Vecchio.

General Description: Located in a renovated fifteenth-century palace which has been divided into seven apartments. The one-room, ground-floor, wheelchair-accessible "Francesco de'Medici" apartment is tastefully furnished, has terracotta floors and vaulted ceilings, and can sleep up to four people. Services include weekly linens, satellite TV, telephone with ISDN access to Internet, independent heating, and air-conditioning. There is a part-time receptionist who speaks English.

Accessibility: There is a portable ramp at the main entrance (one step). Double wooden entrance doors (each 64 centimeters [25 ¼ inches]). Encased doormat. Entrance to apartment is just inside the main door off the vestibule. Width of entrance door to apartment is 95 centimeters (just under 37 ½ inches). Apartment consists of one large room with sitting and dining area, kitchen unit (counters 91 centimeters [35 ¾ inches] high); sleeping area has two single open-frame beds (58 centimeters [22 ¾ inches] high) which can be united to form a double bed. Large couch in sitting area opens into double bed. **Bathroom:** Door (83 centimeters [32 ¾ inches]) opens into spacious area. Tile floor. Ergonomic sink with lever-operated faucet, unwrapped metal pipes. WC (53 centimeters [just under 21 inches] high), adequate space for diagonal and lateral transfer from right (80 centimeters [31 ½ inches]); one retractable grab bar on left. Standard metal wall flush mechanism (120 centimeters [47 ¼ inches] high). Bidet (standard; no grab bars). Alarm cord between sink and WC (too distant from WC). Roll-in shower: 80 centimeters (31 ½ inches) wide. Horizontal grab bars meet at right angles on two walls. Mounted fold-down bench with unpadded seat (32 centimeters [12 ½ inches] wide; 23 centimeters [9 inches] deep) and no armrests is attached to right wall. Lever-operated faucet and removable shower head with hose on wall opposite bench.

Comments: High window next to beds will require assistance for opening and closing, while large window in sitting area is accessible. Shower bench without armrest will be too small and unstable for some users; uncomfortable "reach" for some from the bench to the shower controls on the wall opposite (distance from wall to wall is

80 centimeters [31 ½ inches]). The one alarm cord is too far from the WC (no alarm cord in the shower area). The clothes rack in the wardrobe and the bathroom mirror need to be lowered. The portable ramp at the main entrance must be placed as needed since the street is too narrow to leave it out. Because the receptionist is there only a few hours a day, a wheelchair user will need a companion to deal with the ramp. If you can cope with these few shortcomings, this is a charming place to stay.

Residenza San Gallo
Via San Gallo, 28
50129 Florence
Tel: 055 490 760 or 055 476 622
E-mail: *info@residenzasangallo.com*
Home Page: *www.residenzasangallo.com*

Location: One block west of Piazza San Marco.

General Description: This sunny, one-bedroom, wheelchair-accessible apartment on the *primo piano* (second floor) overlooks a private garden in the heart of Florence. Large L-shaped entry hallway is followed by a combination kitchen, living, dining room. Attractive large bedroom has double bed, and there is an adapted bathroom with a roll-in shower.

Accessibility: Short permanent ramp at main door. Elevator (door width: 73 centimeters [28 ¾ inches]; cabin width: 78 centimeters [30 ¾ inches]; cabin length: 110 centimeters [46 ½ inches]) with raised and Braille signage and audible signal. Apartments No. 1 and No. 2 share an entrance door leading to a short corridor with separate doors to each apartment. Wheelchair-accessible apartment No. 2 has low light switches, remote-controlled thermostat for air-conditioning and heat, TV, intercom system connected to front door downstairs, marble and tile flooring throughout, no telephone. Kitchen is equipped with basic dishes, silverware, pots, and pans. The present dining room table has a base board which makes it unsuitable for wheelchairs. Bedroom has parquet floor; double bed (64 centimeters [25 ¼ inches] high) and slight lip at threshold. Bathroom measures 140 by 260 centimeters (4 feet 7 inches by 8 feet 6 ½ inches). WC (53 centimeters [just under 21 inches] high) has easy-push mechanism, no grab bar. Roll-in shower with flexible hose can be hand held, lever-operated controls, no grab bars, no shower stool. Sink with ergonomic front has lever-operated control, unwrapped metal pipe (with a 29-centimeter [11 ½-inch] clearance under sink), low mirror.

Comments: The gracious owners are willing to accommodate any needs, and exchanging the dining room table, installing a grab bar, or acquiring a chair for the shower should be no problem.

Inexpensive (Under €100)

Hotel Rita Major**
Via della Mattonaia, 43
50121 Florence
Tel: 055 247 7990
Fax: 055 247 8358
E-mail: *info@hotelritamajor.it*
Home Page: *www.hotelritamajor.it*

Location: One block east of Piazza d'Azeglio about a fifteen-minute stroll from Piazza San Marco.

General Description: This is a small (thirty-three rooms) family-run, no-frills hotel with a charming private garden located on a reasonably quiet street. Rooms do not have telephone.

Accessibility: Assistance is required for the step at the front door (10 centimeters [4 inches]), the heavy glass double entrance doors which swing out, and the step down into the garden (12 centimeters [4 ¾ inches]). All interior ground-floor public spaces are accessible.

Double Room No. 14 is a back room on the ground floor with a private door onto the garden (one step down: 20 centimeters [8 inches]). Bathroom is spacious and well appointed with tile floor. Ergonomic sink has wrapped pipe, low mirror. Corner roll-in shower has horizontal grab bars on both walls. WC has handheld bidet shower, retractable grab bar to left, vertical grab bar to right. The main door to the room opens on to a small entrance foyer with two doors: one door leads to the bedroom, the other to the bathroom.

Comments: Next door the *Ristorante Nonna Papera* (with wheelchair-accessible entrance and restroom) serves lunch and dinner at reasonable prices: Via Mattonaia, 51/r, Tel. No: 055 200 1263. Closed all day on Sunday; Friday and Saturday at lunch.

Istituto Gould
Via dei Serragli, 49
50124 Firenze
Tel: 055 212 576
Fax: 055 280 274
Home Page: *www.istitutogould.it*
Office hours and information: 9:00-13:00; 15:00-19:00 except Saturday afternoon and Sunday. No admission of new guests on Saturday afternoons or Sunday.

Location: In the Oltrarno between Piazza Santo Spirito and Piazza del Carmine.

General Description: Situated in a seventeenth-century *palazzo*, this budget accommodation run by the Waldesian church is extremely popular, and reservations to stay there should be made well in advance. There is no curfew since guests are given a key. Meals (including breakfast) are available only for groups of twenty-five or over. Guests are responsible for cleaning their own rooms for the duration of their stay. Three wheelchair-accessible rooms are located on the *primo piano* (second floor) reached by stair lift on the main staircase. **One double (No. 123) and two triples (Nos.**

120 and 121) have private adapted bathrooms with the following features: roll-in shower with mounted fold-down shower bench and grab bars on two walls, WC with fixed grab bar, sink. All rooms are nonsmoking areas.

Accessibility: Sidewalk width in front of entrance door is 110 centimeters (43 ¼ inches). Width of entrance door on street: 80 centimeters (31 ½ inches) with threshold lip of 6 centimeters (2 ³/₈ inches); push door to open. From the main entrance door a corridor leads back to a central courtyard. Width of door to courtyard is 77 centimeters (30 ¼ inches). A portable ramp must be put in place to reach the lift at the base of the staircase and to enter the reception office, both off the courtyard. There is no elevator. The stair lift has a maximum load of 150 kilograms (330 pounds).

Comments: The Isitituto Gould lies ten minutes beyond the Arno in a section of town where the sidewalks tend to be narrow and are often without curb cuts. Wheelchair-accessible Bus D stops on Via Sant'Agostino near the corner of Via dei Serragli, one block down from the Institute. This place is definitely a bargain at €26,00 per person (based on double occupancy; €22,00 per person in a triple). Credit cards accepted. Note: Some power wheelchairs may be too heavy for the stair lift.

Ostello Archi Rossi

Via Faenza, 94r
50123 Firenze
Tel: 055 290 804
Fax: 055 230 2601
Home Page: *www.hostelarchirossi.com*

Location: Two blocks from the railroad station of Santa Maria Novella.

General Description: This no-frills hostel offers dormitory sleeping arrangements for three to nine people per room with two single rooms available on the ground floor near the adapted bathroom. There is a second adapted bathroom upstairs. Services include snack bar, laundry, Internet point, and pay phones, and a hair dryer is available on request. Rooms are cleaned between 11:00 and 14:30, and during this time you may not stay in your room. Curfew is at 2:00 a.m. Towels are provided at small additional cost. Reservations are accepted only from people who are disabled, but you must arrive by 11 a.m. and pay for the room in advance. Rooms are otherwise given out on a "first come, first serve" basis.

Accessibility: There is a ramped entrance at the front door with an internal ramp in the reception area. Doors to single rooms and to adapted bathrooms measure 90 centimeters (35 ½ inches). Bathroom on ground floor has grab bars around WC and roll-in shower. Shower bench is mounted on request. Upstairs bathroom: grab bars in roll-in shower only. Shower space measures 77 centimeter deep by 103 centimeters wide (30 ¼ inches by 40 ½ inches). Shower bench is mounted on request. Elevator to upper floor measures: door: 79 centimeters [31 ¹/₈ inches]); cabin width: 81 centimeters (31 ⁷/₈ inches); cabin length: 129 centimeters (50 ¾ inches). Three steps to the terrace; all other public spaces accessible. Lowered pay telephones.

Comments: Maximum length of stay in this hostel is seven nights, although some exceptions are made. Good location. Generally good accessibility. If you can afford them, the single rooms on the ground floor are the nicest and nearest the more fully adapted bathroom. Price of a dormitory room is €20,00-€23,50 per person, depending on number of beds; €28,50 for a single room. Breakfast and thirty free minutes on Internet are included in the price. Presently credit cards are not accepted, but the management has put in a request to activate this service.

Ostello della Gioventù Villa Camerata
Viale Righi, 2/4
50137 Firenze
Tel: 055 601 451

Fax: 055 610 300
E-mail: *florenceaighostel@virgilio.it*
Home Page: *www.ostellionline.org*
    www.hihostels.org

Location: On the outskirts north of Florence below Fiesole about four kilometers from Piazza San Marco.

General Description: Located in a large villa surrounded by an extensive garden, this youth hostel sleeps over three hundred people in dormitory rooms with bunk beds for four, six, or ten occupants. There is an adapted bathroom on the ground floor with a roll-in shower. Self-service breakfast and dinner are served in two dining rooms with tables also in the garden for outside eating. Ground-floor rooms only are accessible since there is no elevator. Snack bar. Parking. There is a midnight curfew, and you must be out of your room for cleaning between 10:00 and 14:00. You need an international youth hostel card to stay here.

Accessibility: Wheelchair-accessible Bus No. 11 stops a few blocks from the entrance to the villa which is located another six hundred meters (slightly less than $4/10$ miles) up a hill beyond the entrance gate. The unevenly paved asphalt road up to the villa has a fairly steep slope for the first one hundred meters (109 yards) then follows a more gentle incline. Entrance to the villa proper is through a garden with loose gravel paths followed by a ramp onto the villa porch and front door. (You may need assistance to negotiate this because of the gravel deposit at the foot of the ramp.) Only ground-floor rooms are accessible. The adapted bathroom has a roll-in shower with shower bench attached to one of the grab bars. Use with caution as the floor slopes slightly towards center for drainage. WC has a fixed grab bar on left wall and retractable grab bar on the right between the toilet and shower.

Comments: General good accessibility is found once inside the villa, although covering the distance from the nearest accessible bus stop is a challenge. Be sure to request a downstairs room near the accessible bathroom. Price is €16,50 per night, including breakfast.

Youth Firenze 2000
Via Raffaelle Sanzio, 16
50124 Firenze
Tel: 055 233 5558
Fax: 055 230 6392
E-mail: *scatizzi@dada.it*

Location: On the west side of Florence near Ponte della Vittoria across the river from the Cascine Park.

General Description: This is a basic unpretentious place without much character with sixteen rooms located on a raised ground floor reached by a short outside staircase made accessible by stair lift. Rooms have private non-adapted bathrooms (door width to rooms and to private bathrooms: 80 centimeters [31 ½ inches]). There is an adapted bathroom without a shower located in the corridor outside the rooms and an adapted bathroom with a shower in the basement. No meals served, but the breakfast room in the basement has a vending machine selling hot drinks, and free packaged croissants are offered each morning. There is a 2 a.m. curfew. Reservations are advisable.

Description: Wheelchair-accessible Bus No. 12 from the Santa Maria Novella RR station stops 33 meters (36 yards) from the hostel; Wheelchair-accessible Bus No. 13 from Porta Romana stops about 250 meters (273 yards) on the opposite side of street.

Entrance to the hostel is through a reception hall. Threshold step at entrance: 3.5 centimeters (1 ³/₈ inches) up; 9.5 centimeters (3 ¾ inches) down. Exit from the reception hall (threshold lip down 4 centimeters [1 ½ inches]) to an asphalt-paved courtyard, part of which slopes downwards. Most rooms are located on the raised ground-floor level reached by a short external staircase and made accessible by stair lift. There is a short slope down to reach the staircase and stair lift. On the lower basement level (further down the courtyard slope) there is a second adapted bathroom (with roll-in shower) and the breakfast room. The asphalt-paved slope is fairly steep to reach the basement level. A stair lift in the basement is used to reach the level of the bathroom and breakfast room.

Comments: Since this place is not centrally located you must take a bus or taxi to get there. An additional inconvenience is having to go outside your room to the bathroom and taking a shower in the bathroom on the lower level. Assistance is advised for managing the short-but-steep slope in the courtyard. Price of a double-occupancy room is €66,00 with credit cards accepted.

Outside Florence

Hotel owners don't like to admit it, but people are increasingly discovering the advantages of staying outside the city in an apartment in the country, often on a farm or a wine-growing estate. Listed below are three possibilities. Two are located near Tavernelle some 35 kilometers (20 miles) outside Florence; the other, near Impruneta, is 8 kilometers (5 miles) from Porta Romana. Should you want a bucolic setting in the countryside with a swimming pool in an apartment where you have the freedom to fix your own meals without always having to go out to a restaurant to eat, you might consider these possibilities.

La Certaldina
Via Tavolese, 2
Certaldo (Firenze)
Tel: 055 681 5230
Fax: 055 684 161
E-mail: *adriana@tuscanfeeling.it*
Home Page: *www.tuscanfeeling.it*

Location: Approximately halfway between Florence and Siena.

General Description: An attractively furnished, luminous, two-room apartment for a maximum of four people rented for approximately €625,00 per week in high season. Living room, kitchen with sofa bed (sleeps two). Bedroom with double bed. Accessible, adapted bathroom. Swimming pool. Common terrace and sitting area in the *limonia*. A total of eight apartments are presently available for rent in this complex.

Accessibility: The gate to the grounds is normally kept closed, and to open it one must get out of the car and digit a code to open the gate. Digit controls are too high to be reached from the level of a wheelchair. A loose, gravel-covered parking lot is located to the right just inside the entrance gate. Straight ahead is a flagstone driveway leading to the house. A wide, terracotta brick sidewalk from the flagstone driveway takes you directly to the front door of the apartment (approximately 9.50 meters [30 ¾ feet]). Entrance is directly into kitchen area through glass door measuring about 89 centimeters (35 inches). Once you enter the door, you must make a slight turn to the left to enter the main room: space between the entrance door and the end of kitchen counter in the main room is 83 centimeters (32 ⅝ inches). Living room area measures approximately 280 by 480 centimeters (9 ½ by 16 feet) and is attractively furnished with sofa bed, dining table, and chairs. Kitchen counter is 91 centimeters (35 ¾ inches) high. Bedroom has large canopied double bed (58 centimeters [about 22 ¾ inches] high), wardrobe, desk. Window closure is reachable from a wheelchair. Adapted bathroom (230 by 250 centimeters [approximately 7 ½ by 8 feet]) has roll-in shower area with retractable shower seat with two arms and L-shaped grab bar to left (when seated); sink with lever faucet, plastic pipe. WC is 53 centimeters (just under 21 inches) high with retractable grab bar on left and room for right transfer. The route to pool is by wide flagstone path with slight incline (approximately14.50 meters [47 feet] from the corner of the house).

Comments: Owners have recently restructured this comfortable apartment to make it close to being 100 per cent accessible. The present 3.5 centimeter (1 ³/₈ inch) lip at threshold should be adjusted by the time of publication. Easy access to pool, but no pool lift. Possibility to park car near apartment.

Castello Tavolese
Via Tavolese, 71
50052 Certaldo (FI)
Tel: 055 681 5230
Fax: 055 684 161
E-mail: *agriturismo@tavolese.it*
Home Page: *www.tavolese.it*

Location: Between Tavarnelle Val di Pesa and Montespertoli about half an hour's distance from Florence and forty-five minutes from Siena.

General Description: Attractive and well-appointed apartments are located next to a medieval castle in a reconverted farm building on a large wine-growing estate. The wheelchair-accessible apartment *Laudemio* with two bedrooms, a bathroom, a living room-dining room, and a small kitchen is rented year round on a weekly basis for about €1.500. Price includes use of the heated swimming pool, daily cleaning of apartment, daily change of sheets and towels, and breakfast (including farm products: ham and eggs, homemade honey, marmalade, and bread brought to your door each morning).The ground-floor apartment has a private terrace with chairs, tables, and an automatically controlled awning in front of entrance. Living/dining room, with fireplace and satellite TV, measuring 400 by 600 centimeters (13 by 19 ½ feet), is tastefully furnished with some antiques. Kitchenette measures 200 by 200 centimeters (6 ½ by 6 ½ feet). Table linens, porcelain, crystal glasses provided. Large bathroom with ceramic tile floor, tub, roll-in shower, sink, WC, bidet. Corridor between bathroom and bedrooms. Bedrooms measure 400 by 500 centimeters (approximately 12 by 16 ½ feet). In both bedrooms the double beds can be separated.

Description of the Grounds: Driveway is paved with loose gravel. Parking space located near entrance to apartment. Larger parking lot with covered garage located below swimming pool and terrace area. Walkways and poolside terrace paved with smooth terracotta bricks. The pool is situated half inside half outside a converted hay barn with ramp at entrance to inside pool. Inside pool has a raised border of 14 centimeters (5 ½ inches) above floor which is 64 centimeters wide (25 ½ inches)—wide enough for sitting. With ladder, no pool lift. Outside pool is reached by two steps up—first step: 25 centimeters (9 ⁷/₈ inches) high; 33 centimeters (13 inches) deep; second step: 23 centimeters (9 inches) high. Common areas for use of all guests are located near the pool area and include a sitting room with piano, large dining room, accessible restroom (presently without grab bars).Width of door into sitting area: 75 centimeters (29 ½ inches). Dinners can be prepared and served in the dining room for a minimum of twelve guests.

Accessibility: Dining table has knee clearance of 75 centimeters (29 ½ inches). Bathroom has sink with pedestal (difficult frontal approach for large wheelchair). Roll-in shower (dimensions: 76 centimeters [30 inches] deep; 89 centimeters [35 inches] wide), mounted shower bench; vertical and horizontal grab bars. Retractable grab bar and transfer space to left of WC. Height of open-frame beds is 65 centimeters (25 ½ inches).

Comments: Overall very good accessibility in this tasteful and well-appointed apartment. Staff and owners are exceptionally gracious. Five other non-accessible apartments are available for rent in the complex.

Villa il Solatio
Near Mezzamonte
Impruneta (FI)
Tel: 055 234 3354
Fax: 055 234 7240
E-mail: *info@pitcherflaccomio.com*
Home Page: *www.pitcherflaccomio.com*

Location: About eight kilometers (five miles) south of Florence near Mezzamonte on the way to Impruneta.

General Description: This attractive two-story apartment has been renovated for wheelchair use. Entry is from the garden into the dining area. There are also a large living room, a separate eat-in kitchen, and two bathrooms (one wheelchair accessible) on the ground floor. A staircase (twenty steps) without handrail and elevator lead to three upstairs bedrooms and bath. Hardwood, terracotta, and tile floors are throughout. The apartment is equipped with telephone, three TVs, VCR, stereo, dishwasher, and washing machine. Outside seating area in garden has table and chairs. A swimming pool is located on the grounds. There is parking space for two cars. Weekly rental is between €850 (low season) and €1.650 (high season).

Accessibility: Driveway and parking area have new asphalt pavement. There is a slight slope up to the level of the lawn in front of the house. Flagstone path leads to entrance with two steps. Ramp available. Double doors; both need to be opened to permit passage of wheelchair. Wheelchair-accessible downstairs bathroom measures 280 by 180 centimeters (9 feet 2 ¼ inches by 5 feet 11 inches) and has roll-in shower with flexible hose which can be hand held. No shower bench. Pedestal sink with short-lever faucet. WC: 46 centimeters (18 inches) high; no grab bars. Elevator door measures 75 centimeters (29 ½ inches); cabin width: 100 centimeters (39 ³/₈ inches); cabin length: almost 95 centimeters (just under 37 ½ inches). Upstairs bathroom door measures 68 centimeters (26 ¾ inches); large bathroom measures 300 by 220 centimeters (9 feet 10 inches by 7 feet 2 ½ inches) and has box shower with a 16-centimeter (6 ¼-inch) base edge; WC (no grab bars), sink, and bidet. First bedroom has double bed (can be separated) 57 centimeters (22 ½ inches) high; second bedroom has an antique double bed (66 centimeters [26 inches] high) with a solid wooden pedestal base. Third bedroom with small twin beds (47 centimeters [18 ½ inches] high) is more suitable for children.

Comments: The owners live on the property and share the pool which is not accessible to wheelchairs (six steps and a rough flagstone walk lead to the pool). While there is the inconvenience of having to go downstairs to take a shower and not being able to get to the pool (somewhat compensated by the lovely views) all in all, this place has decent accessibility, tried and tested by the owner's wife who used a wheelchair and once lived in the house. Should you require a shower chair, it can be provided. The recently relocated Coop supermarket in nearby Impruneta is wheelchair accessible, as is the new Ristorante/Pizzeria "Il Pruneto" (with wheelchair-accessible restroom) above the supermarket.

Places to Eat

Eating in Italy is more than a national pastime; it's almost a sacred rite, and it's not surprising to find that the international Slow Food Movement, now with offices in New York City, began in 1986 in Italy. Each Italian region has its specialties, and the traditional dishes found in Florence are entirely different from those found in Naples or Rome. Simple, hardy, and down-to-earth, many Florentine dishes derive from peasant fare: *panzanella*, made from crusty old bread soaked in water and flavored with oil and vinegar, tomatoes, onions, and cucumber; *ribollita* (bread and vegetable soup) or *pappa al pomodoro* (bread soup with tomatoes). The secret of Florentine cooking lies in the first-rate quality of its ingredients. *Fettunta* is nothing more than good Tuscan bread toasted and seasoned with garlic and olive oil. November's freshly pressed pungent olive oil is best. Nothing could be simpler than *pecorino con le pere,* pears eaten with cheese made from sheep's milk, whose popularity is understood by the old saying: *al contadino non far' sapere quant'è buono il cacio con le pere* (don't tell the farmer how good his *pecorino* tastes with pears, otherwise he won't give it up!)

Probably Florence can be best described as a "meat-and-potatoes town." Typical meat dishes include *bistecca alla fiorentina,* a T-bone steak coming from the Chianina breed of cattle or *spezzatino,* stewed beef. Pork, tripe, rabbit, chicken, and guinea fowl, cooked in a variety of ways, regularly appear on the tables of both Florentine households and *trattorie.*

Food in Italy is often subject to the changing seasons. What you find sold in a Florentine bakery is a good example. *Cenci* (rags), a sweet, crisp fried batter, suddenly appear on the Thursday before Shrove Tuesday; *schiacciata alla fiorentina,* a sponge cake decorated with powdered sugar, throughout the Carnival season preceding Lent. Around Easter time you'll find *pan di ramerino,* a rosemary-flavored bun, and on March 19 for the feast day of San Giuseppe and for a short period after, *frittelle di riso* (rice fritters). With the wine harvest in September, the traditional sweet is *schiacciata con l'uva,* a pastry made with wine (not table) grapes, followed in November by *castagnaccio,* a flat chestnut flour cake made with rosemary and pine nuts. *Panettone,* a cake with raisins and candied fruit, appears at Christmas.

Another good indication of how much Italians appreciate food can be seen by the number of different kinds of places where you can eat. In a *pizzeria* you will find pizza, often in addition to pasta and main course dishes. A *rosticceria* serves roast chicken, pork, roast beef, and numerous vegetable and pasta dishes and, though often just a take-out service, may sometimes have tables. A *tavola calda* has ready-made dishes and is often set up cafeteria style. An *osteria* in the old days was an inn offering both food and lodging. Today it is more like a *trattoria,* which is usually, *but not always,* a simple, unpretentious restaurant. A restaurant or *ristorante* used to imply a more formal atmosphere with waiters dressed in white jackets and tables set with linen napkins and tablecloths. Today the distinctions between an *osteria,* a *trattoria,* and a *ristorante* are not always so clear. Bars, unlike in the USA, do not serve exclusively alcoholic beverages and are really more like *cafés,* though a bar may sometimes only have a stand-up counter, while a café will have tables for seating. In both bars and *cafés* you can always find something to eat: an assortment of pastries or sandwiches, known as *panini* or *tramezzini* (sandwiches which are triangular shaped), "toast" (sliced ham and cheese on toasted bread), and sometimes salad and pasta plates. An *enoteca,* instead, is a wine store which sometimes also serves things to eat.

A few words of advice for eating out in Italy: If you enter a traditional *ristorante* or *trattoria* you are usually expected to commit yourself to a full meal. An Italian might start with an antipasto, followed by a first course or *primo,* usually a pasta, rice, or soup dish. The main course or *secondo* follows: meat or fish accompanied by a vegetable (*contorno*) or a salad (*insalata*). Fruit (*frutta*), cheese (*formaggio*), or dessert (*dolce*), some coffee and even a final *digestivo* (a special liqueur to help digest all that food) can end the meal. The meal is accompanied by wine and bottled water (water from the tap is almost never served). If you cannot handle so much food, you can order less. For example, skip the antipasto and have a pasta, followed by a main dish (or skip the pasta and have the antipasto instead). The waiters will usually understand if you want to substitute the meat course with a vegetable or with cheese and a salad. These shortcuts are acceptable as long as you order several dishes and not just a single plate. However, you'll also find that in cities that cater to tourists like Florence, some places are beginning to follow a new trend in offering single-plate meals at lunchtime. For a one-plate meal you could also go to a *tavola calda* or to a bar or café that serve sandwiches, pasta, and salads. A few such "one plate" places are the **Ristorante Finisterrae** in Piazza Santa Croce, **Cantinetta da Verrazzano** near Piazza Signoria, or the cafés in Piazza della Repubblica.

Eating out is popular in Florence, and you should always make sure to make a reservation. Be sure to explain if you are in a wheelchair so that you will be given a table that is comfortable for you and, if necessary, receive help at the entrance to the restaurant. In general, one has lunch in Italy between 12:30 and 14:00 and dinner between 19:30 and 22:30.

The following list has been divided geographically into neighborhoods, with a brief section at the end concerning places serving gluten-free meals. The basis of criteria for inclusion in the first part is a wheelchair-accessible locale, sometimes with outside seating only, usually with a wheelchair-accessible restroom or, if not, with a wheelchair-accessible restroom nearby. A few bars serving sandwiches or simple *primi* have also been mentioned. In general, attention has been given to indicate certain characteristics of each place: if the food is noteworthy or not, if the clientele are primarily tourists or Florentines, or if the bill will be particularly steep. Many places in Florence, especially in the piazzas, will have outside seating, weather permitting, from around the middle of March to around the middle of November, offering further options for accessibility.

From the Duomo to Piazza della Signoria

Al Lume di Candela
Via delle Terme, 23/r
Tel: 055 265 6561
Open: Monday-Saturday, 12:00-14:30; 19:30-23:00; closed on Sunday

This attractive new place is located between Piazza della Signoria and Via Tornabuoni. There is one **high step** (17 centimeters [6 ¾ inches]) at the entrance from a narrow sidewalk (36 centimeters [14 ¹/₈ inches] wide) with a 6-centimeter (2 ³/₈-inch) curb; doorbell to call for assistance. **Accessible restroom** with transfer space and retractable grab bar to right of WC; vertical grab bar placed near wall on left.

Antico Fattore
Via Lambertesca, 1/r
Tel: 055 288 975
Open: 12:00-15:00; 19:30-22:30; closed on Sunday

With accessible entrance, located near the Uffizi, **no accessible restroom**, but it's a traditional Florentine *trattoria*, visited by the president of Italy when he's in town. Also has a vegetarian menu. The nearest public restroom is in Via Filippina on the way to Santa Croce (see chapter on "Santa Croce" for location).

Cafeteria degli Uffizi
Galleria degli Uffizi
Tel: 335 310 366
Open: 9:30-18:00 except Monday when the museum is closed

The cafeteria is found in the west wing on the top floor where the main galleries are located, has an outside terrace, and serves the standard sandwiches, ice cream, pastries, and *primi*. There is a platform lift at the entrance and an **accessible restroom** close by in the west wing of the museum.

Cantinetta dei Verrazzano

Via de' Tavolini, 18-20/r

Tel: 055 268 590

Open: Monday-Saturday, 8:00-21:00; lunch 12:30-14:30; closed on Sunday and two weeks in August

With a bakery up front and marble-topped tables in the back for eating, this is the place for a morning *cappuccino* and pastry or a lunchtime sandwich and a glass of wine. *Cantinetta* means little wine cellar and refers to the bottles of Verrazzano wine from the owners' family vineyards, which is also for sale here. **Accessible restroom** has retractable grab bar with transfer space to right of WC and a vertical grab bar to the left.

Hot Pot

Via Vacchereccia, 3/r

Tel: 055 2 302 396

Open: 10:00-23:30; closed on Monday

This self-service cafeteria, right off Piazza della Signoria, may be short on charm and atmosphere, but it's a good solution for a quick and relatively inexpensive bite to eat. One **low step at entrance:** 7 centimeters (2 ¾ inches). Outside seating. **Accessible restroom** with retractable grab bar on right. Limited transfer space.

I Buongustai

Via dei Cerchi, 15/r

Tel: 055 291 304

Open: Monday-Thursday, 8:00-19:30; Friday-Saturday 8:00-22:30; closed on Sunday and part of August

Located just off Piazza della Signoria, this is an informal place to eat pasta and salad dishes, cold cuts, and *bruschette* or toasted bread served with a variety of toppings. Some daily special meat dishes are offered as well. There is a **ramp at the entrance** which is narrowed by stools at the counter near the door. Suitable for small manual wheelchairs. Small **accessible restroom** with grab bar and room for left transfer.

I Fratellini
Via dei Cimatori, 38/r
Tel: 055 239 6096
Open: Monday-Saturday, 8:00-19:00; closed on most Sunday and in August

I Fratellini has been a Florentine standby long before fast-food operations came to town. Try it for a quick glass of wine and a *panino* (sandwich) bought over a sidewalk counter and eaten on the street together with the locals. Sidewalk curb. No seating. **No restroom.**

La Grotta Guelfa
Via Pellicceria, 5/r
Tel: 055 210 042
Open: Every day 12:00-14:30; 19:00-22:30

There are tables inside and outside under the loggia, lots of tourists and an **accessible restroom** (no grab bars, low WC) downstairs in the basement (elevator). Go to the end of the left porch for easiest access (4-centimeter [1 ½-inch] rise). Tends to serve on into the afternoon after other places have closed.

L'Incontro
Hotel Savoy
Piazza della Repubblica, 7
Tel: 055 273 5891
Open: 12:30-14:30; 19:30-22:30

This *bar/ristorante*, part of the Savoy Hotel, serves Tuscan and international cuisine, has outside and inside seating, and as one would expect of a five-star deluxe hotel, is expensive. **Accessible restroom** in the basement with elevator large enough for a scooter.

La Terrazza
La Rinascente
Piazza della Repubblica, 1
Tel: 055 283 612
Open: Monday-Saturday, 10:00-21:00; Sunday 10:30-20:00

An outdoor rooftop terrace bar/café with a spectacular view located in the department store La Rinascente. Light lunch is served from 12:00 to 15:00, the usual snacks and *panini*, anytime. It's also a place where you can go in the evening for a drink (*aperitivo*). In case of rain, there is a bar on the mezzanine level below with more difficult accessibility due to some tables and chairs placed too close to the elevator. To operate the elevator, you must keep the button pushed in until you reach the terrace. Elevator dimensions are door width: 89 centimeters (35 inches); cabin length: 115 centimeters (45 ¼ inches). There is an **accessible restroom** on the top floor in the southeast corner of the store. Restroom has horizontal and vertical grab bars to the right of the WC (height: 51 centimeters [20 inches]) with transfer space from left.

Robiglio
Via Tosinghi, 11/r
Tel: 055 215 013
Open: Monday-Saturday, 8:00-20:00

A popular spot for coffee and pastries, this *pasticceria* also serves a sit-down lunch. There is one low step (6 centimeters [2 ³/₈ inches]) at the entrance to the bar in Via Tosinghi (doorbell). The entrance to the lunchroom is through the big arched doorway to the left in Via Tosinghi. A **ramp** will be placed at this door upon request. **Accessible restroom** has fixed grab bar to right of WC.

Ristorante/Pizzeria Il Bargello
Piazza della Signoria, 4/r
Tel: 055 214 071
Open: 12:00-22:30; closed on Monday

A large restaurant, with both outside and inside seating, catering to tourists and groups. Hospitable atmosphere. Offers gluten-free menu. **Threshold step:** 10 centimeters (4 inches), but management has assured that a ramp has been ordered. Once inside the door there is a narrow corridor (78 centimeters [30 ¾ inches]) before reaching the dining room. Well-maintained **accessible restroom** with fixed grab bar to left, retractable grab bar to right of WC.

Trattoria Da Pennello
Via Dante Alighieri 4/r
Tel: 055 294 848
Open: Tuesday-Saturday, lunch and dinner; Sunday, lunch only

Typical Tuscan *trattoria*. Moderately expensive. They do have guests coming in wheelchairs, but the entrance is tricky and will require assistance: **one low step:** 8 centimeters (3 ⅛ inches); door: 67 centimeters (just under 26 ½ inches) wide; ramp inside entrance. **No accessible restroom.** The nearest public restroom is in Via Filippina on the way to Santa Croce (see chapter on "Santa Croce" for location).

Uffizi Center
Piazza del Grano (behind the Uffizi at the top of Via de' Neri)
Open: Everyday from 8:00-2:00 a.m. (bar); 10:00-22:00 (shops and restaurant)
E-mail: *info@uffizicenter.com*
Home Page: *www.uffizicenter.com*

The bar on the ground floor, with tables inside and outside on the loggia, also serves light meals. The restaurant upstairs is self-service at lunchtime with full service for the evening meal. In between are two floors of shops selling typical Florentine crafts. A wheelchair accessible restroom is located on the basement level (WC 47 centimeters [18 ½ inches] high with retractable grab bar on right. Transfer from right is somewhat impeded by the position of the grab bar. No left transfer). Fee: €0,60. Elevator serves all floors (door width: 80 centimeters [31 ½ inches]; cabin width: 110 centimeters [43 ¼ inches]; cabin length: 137 centimeters [54 inches]). Wheelchair-accessible entrance is located in Via del Castello d'Altafronte (street to the left of the loggia entrance) through automatic doors with a slight threshold lip. Sidewalk is lowered at the loggia end with a 7 centimeter (2 ¾ inch) curb in front of the door. There is another wheelchair-accessible restroom reached by stair lift on the 3rd floor (2° *piano*).

Outdoor Cafés

Piazza della Signoria
Most places on the piazza have outside seating from mid-March to November and are accessible from the sidewalk. Only the Ristorante Il Bargello and the Hot Pot Cafeteria have accessible restrooms.

Rivoire
Piazza della Signoria 5/r
Tel: 055 211 302
Open: 8:00-24:00; closed on Monday

Rivoire is a Florentine landmark, famous for its chocolate, quite expensive if you sit at a table, less so if you take something directly at the bar. **No accessible restroom.** (The nearest accessible restroom is in the Palazzo Vecchio, although in order to use it in theory you should have a ticket for the museum.)

Piazza della Reppublica
The cafés in Piazza della Repubblica are a Florentine institution and have been around since the nineteenth century. All serve breakast, lunch, and dinner and have inside seating but are also popular places for a

quick espresso or a late-afternoon aperitivo. None have accessible restrooms, but the Hotel Savoy and the department store La Rinascente on the east side of the piazza do.

Gilli

Piazza della Repubblica, 39/r
Tel: 055 213 896
Open: Monday, Wednesday-Sunday, 7:30-24:00; closed on Tuesday

Outside seating accessible from sidewalk. One **step at entrance**. **No accessible restroom**.

Giubbe Rosse

Piazza della Repubblica, 13/r
Tel: 055 290 052
Open: Monday-Tuesday, Thursday-Sunday, 8:00-24:00; closed on Wednesday

Outside seating accessible from sidewalk. One **step at entrance**. **No accessible restroom**.

Paszkowski

Piazza della Repubblica, 31-35/r
Open: Tuesday-Sunday, 7:00-1:30 a.m; closed on Monday

Ramp from piazza to outside seating. One **step at main entrance**. **No accessible restroom**.

Bars serving sandwiches

Caffè Duomo

Piazza del Duomo, 34/r
Tel: 055 211 348
Open: 8:00-24:00 seven days a week

Located on the north side of the Duomo, with **accessible restroom**.

Other

Tripe vendor in Piazza del Mercato Nuovo. This open stand selling sandwiches and both hot and cold tripe and *lampredotto* dishes has a low counter (wheelchair height) on which to perch your food and drink.

Santa Maria Novella

Coco Lezzone
Via del Parioncino, 26/r (near Palazzo Rucellai)
Tel: 055 287 178
Open: Monday, Wednesday-Saturday; lunch and dinner; Tuesday, lunch; closed on Sunday

Popular *trattoria*, frequented by Florentines and tourists alike, serving hearty Tuscan food at expensive prices. **One step** (10 centimeters [4 inches]) with a 10-centimeter (4-inch) curb on the sidewalk in front of the entrance. (Power wheelchairs have been known to enter this restaurant.) **No accessible restroom.**

Il Latini
Via dei Palchetti, 6/r
Tel: 055 210 916
Open: 12:30-14:30; 19:30-22:30; closed on Monday

You always need a reservation to get into this popular, crowded *trattoria*; everyone seems to know about it. Can't be beat for genuine Tuscan cooking and atmosphere. Moderately expensive. **Accessible restroom.**

La Rotonda
Via il Prato, 10-16/r
Tel: 055 265 4644
Open: Every day, 18:00-2:00 a.m.; closed part of August

A big, noisy place to drink beer and eat pizza. Popular with the younger crowd. **Accessible restroom** with fixed vertical and horizontal grab bars to right of WC, transfer space to left.

MacDonald's
Via Valfonda, 25/r (ramp at entrance; no doorbell)
Tel: 055 282 885
Open: Every day, 8:00-4:00 a.m.; Friday and Saturday, twenty-four hours

Accessible restroom in basement. WC has transfer space to left, vertical grab bar to right. You will have to ask to be accompanied there in the elevator.

Marione
Via della Spada, 27/r
Tel: 055 214 756
Open: Every day, 12:00-15:00; 19:00-22:30

Informal *trattoria* with home-style cooking. Lots of locals. No accessible restroom. Five-centimeter (2-inch) threshold lip at entrance.

Osteria N. 1
Via del Moro, 18-20
Tel: 055 284 897
Open: Monday-Saturday, 12:00-15:00; 18:00-24:00; closed on Sunday

An attractive place serving Tuscan-Venetian cuisine. One step at the entrance (7 centimeters [2 ¾ inches]) from a narrow sidewalk with a 12-centimeter (4 ¾-inch) curb. Moderately expensive. Accessible restroom with transfer space to right of WC; fixed grab bar on left wall.

San Lorenzo

Da Garibaldi
Piazza del Mercato Centrale, 38/r
Tel: 055 212 267
Home Page: *www.garibaldi.it*
Open: Every day, 11:30-23:00

Friendly atmosphere with traditional Tuscan cooking. One step up to outside seating. Inside has several small dining rooms. One step up to nonsmoking area. Decent **accessible restroom** with vertical grab bar near right wall and slightly in front of the WC, retractable grab bar to left. You may have to ask them to move the baby-changing table.

Spleen Café
Borgo San Lorenzo 31/r
Tel: 055 287 481
Open: High season, 10:30-22:30; low season, 11:30-15:30 and 17:30-1:30 a.m.

A no-frills, self-service restaurant with **ramp at entrance**, accessible route to dining areas, and **accessible restroom** (WC has grab bars and room for right transfer).

La Gratella
Via Guelfa, 81
Tel: 055 211 292
Open: 12:00-15:00; 19:00-23:00

Pleasant small *trattoria* serving standard Tuscan cuisine located a few blocks west of Via Nazionale near Piazza Indipendenza. Also has a gluten-free menu. The front room is accessible to wheelchairs; two steps to garden and rear dining room. **Accessible restroom** has sliding doors and retractable grab bar to left of WC.

Nannini
Borgo San Lorenzo, 7/r
Tel: 055 212 680
Open: Every day, 7:30-20:15

A bar/*tavola calda* serving the usual sandwiches, salad plates, and pasta dishes. Specialty: sweets from Siena. Usually crowded. **Accessible restroom** with fixed grab bar to left, retractable grab bar and transfer space to right of WC.

Nerbone
Mercato Centrale di San Lorenzo
Tel: 055 219 949
Open: Monday-Saturday, 7:00-14:00; closed on Sunday

Market workers, tourists, and Florentines flock here for sandwich, often tripe, and a glass of wine. It's a rowdy, colorful informal place where you have to elbow your way up to the counter to order. There is one step up to the places to sit. There is an **accessible restroom in the southwest corner of the market.**

Za Za
Piazza del Mercato Centrale, 26/r
Tel: 055 215 411
Open: Lunch and dinner; closed on Sunday

A popular neighborhood place which has been serving classic Tuscan dishes for years. One step up to outside seating. The somewhat-crowded interior is accessible through the door to the right of the main entrance. There is a ramp to the miniscule restroom which is not accessible to wheelchairs. **Around the corner in Via della Stufa, 25, there is a public, accessible restroom** open until 18:00 (19:00 during the summer. In 2003 the restroom was open until midnight in August and September).

San Marco

Buffet Freddo
Via Alfani 70/r
Open: 9:00-16:30; closed on Sunday

A very informal tiny locale around the corner from the Accademia serving delicious, typical straightforward Florentine food. You order at the counter, and the food is brought to the table. To avoid the rush, and sometimes just to get in the door, don't go between 12:30 and 14:00. Level entrance. **No restroom.**

Il Vegetariano
Via delle Ruote, 30/r
Tel: 055 475 030
Open: Tuesday-Friday, 12:30-14:00; 19:30-22:30; Saturday and
Sunday, 19:30-22:30

This self-service vegetarian eatery has been highly popular since it opened in the 1970s. It has one **step at the entrance** and a short, steep ramp down to the back dining area and to the **accessible restroom (no grab bars)**.

McDonald's
Via Cavour, 61/r
Tel: 055 294 105
Open: Every day, 10:00-22:00; Friday, Saturday, Sunday, until 23:00

Florence resisted for years but finally ceded to fast food. **Accessible restroom** (with fixed grab bar to right of WC).

Nabbucco Wine Bar
Via XXVII Aprile, 28/r
Tel: 055 475 087
Open: 6:30-22:00; closed Sunday

Located across the street from the Cenacolo di Sant'Apollonia, this place with one **step at the entrance** (11 centimeters [4 ¼ inches]) serves breakfast, lunch (an assortment of sandwiches, salad, cheese, and pasta dishes) and drinks and light supper in the evening. The accessible entrance, just around the corner in Via S. Reparata, has a short ramp but is kept locked, and you will have to request that it be opened. To reach the **accessible restroom** you have to pass through a set of narrow "Western style" swinging doors (approximately 65 centimeters [just over 25 ½ inches] wide).

Ristorante/ Wine Bar Semidivino
Via San Gallo 22/r
Tel: 055 462 0016
Open: Every day between 11:00 and 24:00

Features of this informal restaurant include Tuscan cuisine, a nonsmoking room, outside seating. **One step at entrance** (approximately 16.5 centimeters [6 ½ inches]) and an **accessible restroom** (vertical grab bar on left wall; transfer space on right).

Santa Croce

Caffè Pasticceria La Loggia degli Albizi
Borgo degli Albizzi, 39/r
Tel: 055 247 9574
Open: Monday-Saturday, 7:00-20:00; closed on Sunday

You can stop here for a morning or afternoon coffee and pastry or for an assortment of pasta and salad dishes at lunchtime. The wheelchair-accessible entrance is from the small piazza to the side. **Ramp** is steep, and sidewalk in front of entrance has no curb cut. Their **restroom is accessible** but, on the day of inspection, was crowded with cleaning equipment, and the seat on the WC was missing.

Da Benvenuto
Via della Mosca 16/r (corner of Via de'Neri)
Tel: 055 214 833
Open: Monday-Saturday, 12:00-14:30; 19:00-22:30; closed on Sunday

You'll find a noisy mix of neighborhood locals and tourists in this *trattoria* which serves unpretentious Florentine food at affordable prices. **Ramp at entrance. Accessible restroom without grab bars.**

Dantè
Via Giovanni da Verrazzano, 5/r
Tel: 055 244 528
Open: Monday-Saturday, lunch, 12:00-15:00; 19:00-22:30; closed on Saturday evening and on Sunday

This inexpensive small *trattoria*, with an emphasis on Tuscan cooking, is located just north of Piazza Santa Croce, but despite its location two steps off the beaten path, few tourists seem to have discovered it. **No accessible restroom.** There is a public restroom on the other side of the piazza in Borgo Santa Croce, 29/r next to the tourist information office.

Da Rocco
Inside the Mercato di Sant'Ambrogio
Open: Monday-Saturday, 12:00-14:30

An informal, friendly, and inexpensive *tavola calda* right in the middle of the market building. Good place for a quick bite to eat. Market workers and local shoppers share tables grouped around the edge of a common central serving area attached to a small kitchen. Although the built-in tables with benches are high, a wheelchair can still roll up to the end of one of them. The "accessible" **public restroom in the basement** is very cramped, suitable for small manual wheelchairs only.

Finisterrae
Piazza Santa Croce, 12
Tel: 055 263 8675
Open: Every day, 11:30-14:00; 19:30-23:30

This restaurant features a wide variety of Mediterranean dishes ranging from falafel and tabouleh, to paella, moussaka, and bistecca alla fiorentina. The room in the back overlooking the garden is the nicest. Tables are nicely spaced, and there is an **accessible restroom,** quite large with fixed grab bar on left wall and retractable bar on right. Short **ramp at entrance.**

Gusto Leo
Via del Proconsolo 8-10/r
Tel: 055 285 217
Open: Every day, 8:00-1 a.m.

Informal, no-frills eatery with convenient location just down the street from the Bargello Museum and on the way to the Duomo. Offers a wide variety of things to eat and has an **accessible restoom** with fixed bar to right of WC; retractable grab bar and transfer space on the left.

Pizzeria/ Ristorante I Ghibellini
Piazza San Pier Maggiore 8/9/10
Tel: 055 214 424
Open: Monday-Tuesday, Thursday-Sunday 12:00-16:00; 19:00-1:00 a.m.; closed on Wednesday

Located in an old fourteenth-century palazzo, I Ghibellini offers classic Tuscan cuisine and a large choice of fifty different kinds of pizza. One **high step at entrance** (18 centimeters [about 7 inches]). **Accessible restroom** with transfer space on left side of WC and fixed grab bar on right wall.

Ristorante Cibreo
Via Andrea del Verrocchio, 8/r
Tel: 055 234 1100
Open: Tuesday-Saturday, 13:00-14:30; 19:00-23:00

Cibreo is another one of those famous places that everyone knows about. The cuisine and the service are innovative variations on a Tuscan theme. Expensive. **One step at entrance. Accessible restroom** (WC with grab bars).

Trattoria Accadi
Via Borgo Pinti, 56/r
Tel: 055 247 8410
Open: Monday-Saturday, lunch and dinner; closed on Sunday

This is an unpretentious *trattoria* offering Tuscan cooking. There is an **accessible restroom** off the second dining room: one step down (10 centimeters [4 inches]). Transfer space to right of WC; fixed grab bar on left wall.

Oltrarno

Café in Palazzo Pitti.
Open: During museum hours

Serves light lunch and snacks. There is an **accessible restroom in the courtyard** of palace next to the café.

Golden View Open Bar
Via dei Bardi 58/r
Tel: 055 214 502
Open: Daily, 11:30-2:00 a.m.

Located near the Ponte Vecchio just off the beaten track to the Pitti Palace museums, this new combination *ristorante*, wine bar, and *pizzeria* seems to be geared for tourists. Has live jazz Monday and Wednesday nights at 21:00 and great views of the river. **Accessible restroom** with fixed grab bar to left of WC, retractable grab bar and room for transfer to right.

Il Santo Bevitore
Via Santo Spirito, 64-66/r
Tel: 055 211 264
Open: 12:00-14:30; 19:30-23:30; closed on Sunday

Brick-vaulted ceilings and lots of space in this casual wine bar serving assorted salads, cheese plates, and *primi*. **Level entrance.**

The large **accessible restroom** has transfer space from the left side with one vertical grab bar placed in front of the WC on the right.

O!o
Piazza Piattellina 7/r
Tel: 055 212 917
Open: 10:00-1:30 a.m.; closed on Monday

Informal place serving breakfast, lunch, and dinner. **Accessible restroom.** WC has fixed grab bar on left wall with transfer space on right.

Trattoria Quattro Leoni
Via de' Vellutini 1/r
Tel: 055 218 562
Open: 12:00-14:30; 19:00-23:00

Friendly, usually crowded place with **accessible outside seating.** Entrance not accessible to wheelchairs: one step onto sidewalk from the level of the piazza (10 centimeters [4 inches]), second step (10 centimeters [4 inches]) through door (width: 76 centimeters [30 ½ inches]). **No accessible restroom,** but if you're there for lunch, there is the **accessible public restroom nearby in Via dello Sprone.** Moderately expensive. Reservations advised especially for outside seating.

Ristorante and Bar Ricchi
Piazza Santo Spirito, 8/r
Tel: 055 215 864
Open: 12:30-15:00; 19:30-23:00 (restaurant); 7:00-21:00 (bar-stays open until 1:30 a.m. during high season); closed on Sunday

This small restaurant serves typical Tuscan dishes for lunch; fish only at dinner. Reservations at dinner advised. At the bar you can get anything from ice cream to sandwiches and assorted *primi*. Seating is available outside (one step); there are several steps into the seating area near the bar. Level entrance for dining room and bar. **Accessible restroom** through bar area (fixed grab bar to left of WC, transfer space to right). The ramp into restroom is somewhat steep, but manageable.

Ristorante/Wine Bar Beccofino
Piazza degli Scarlatti, 1/r (Lungarno Guicciardini)
Tel: 055 290 076
Open: Tuesday-Sunday, 19:30-23:30; Sunday, lunch, 12:30-14:30

Popular and stylish restaurant with innovative cooking which is modern like the decor. The wine bar has a lighter menu. Outside seating in warm weather. Expensive. **One low step at entrance** to the restaurant: 9 centimeters (3 ½ inches); ring doorbell for assistance. **Accessible restroom** (WC has fixed horizontal grab bar to left, transfer space to right. Unprotected metal pipe under sink). One step to reach the restroom from the wine bar area but not from the restaurant.

Outside the City Walls

Trattoria Donnini
Via di Rimaggio, 22
Bagno a Ripoli
Tel: 055 630 076.
Closed: All day Wednesday and Thursday lunch

An elegant small restaurant located about three miles southeast of Florence. Menu offers local ingredients cooked in an innovative way. Expensive. **Low ramp at entrance.** Ramps within interior allow access to both dining rooms. **Accessible restroom** has retractable grab bar to left of WC, transfer space to right. The accessible entrance to the garden, set up with tables in late spring, summer, and early fall, is located off the driveway. Parking available.

Trattoria Zibibbo
Via di Terzollina, 3/r (near the Careggi Hospital)
Tel: 055 433 383

Open: Monday-Saturday, 12:30-15:30; 19:30-24:00; closed on Sunday and in August

Food is cooked with the best ingredients in this exceptionally attractive and innovative *trattoria* offering Tuscan and Sicilian dishes sometimes with a Middle Eastern influence. There is an **accessible restroom** without grab bars and **two steps at the entrance** (each about 15 centimeters [6 inches] high). After the first step from the street there is space for a wheelchair to approach the second step at the door, and the staff is more than willing to give a hand. Expensive. The owner also conducts a cooking school here.

Ristorante/Pizzeria Il Pruneto
Via della Croce, 39 (next to the Casa del Popolo)
Impruneta
Tel: 055 231 4760
Open: seven days a week (except in November when closed Mondays), 12:00-14:30; 19:00-24:00

Located in a lovely little town to the south of Florence about a twenty minute drive from Porta Romana, this new restaurant offers pizza on Thursday for lunch and every evening and has a fixed price menu at in the middle of the day for lunch. Innovative Tuscan cooking. There is outside seating from June to October on a roof top terrace with sweeping views of the Tuscan countryside. Both the **roof top terrace and restroom are accessible to wheelchairs.** WC has fixed grab bar on right wall, retractable grab bar on left with room for left transfer. The restaurant also offers courses in cooking and wine tasting.

Ristorante La Loggia
Piazzale Michelangelo,1
Tel: 055 234 2832 or 234 5288
Closed: Monday

Also has a bar/café serving sandwiches. Expensive but with a spectacular view of the city below. In nice weather you can sit outside. **Entrance with ramp** onto the loggia at the left end of the loggia towards the parking lot. Note: Call ahead of time so that waiter will know to move the potted plant placed at the top of the ramp. **Accessible restroom** has fixed grab bar to left of WC, retractable bar to right but no space for side transfer.

Gluten-free Meals

For further information, including a list of restaurants throughout Italy which serve gluten-free food as well as suggestions from the National Italian Celiac Association of how to choose what to eat when in Italy, see *www.celiachia.it.*

In addition to **Ristorante/Pizzeria Il Bargello** and **Trattoria La Gratella** listed above, the following places offering gluten-free menus, are fairly centrally located and are approved by the National Celiac Association:

Enotria
Via delle Porte Nuove, 50 (just outside Porta a Prato)
Tel: 055 354 350
Open: Monday-Saturday, 12:00-15:30; 19:30-midnight; closed on Monday evening and Sunday

A wine shop serving food. From the *antipasti* to the dessert, there is a recommendation for which wine to drink with each dish. Moderately expensive.

Ristorante Al Tranvai
Piazza Tasso 14/r (near Piazza del Carmine)
Tel: 055 225 197
Open: Monday-Friday, 12:00-14:30; 19:15-22:45

It's a squeeze into this popular place serving traditional Florentine food.

Ristorante I Quattro Amici
Via Orto Oricellari, 29 (near the RR station)
Tel: 055 215 413
Open: 12:00-14:30; 19:00-22:30; Closed on Sunday

Specialty: fish

Il Portale
Via Alamanni, 29/r (near the RR station)
Tel: 055 212 992
Open: 7:00-midnight (bar); 12:00-14:30; 19:00-22:30

Specialty: pizza in the evening

Ristorante Targa Bistrot Caffè Concerto
Lungarno Colombo, 7 (between Ponte San Niccolò and Ponte da Verrazzano)
Tel: 055 677 377
Open: Monday-Saturday, 12:30-14:30; 20:00-22:45; closed on Sunday

An attractive restaurant on the banks of the Arno, beyond the *viali* and east of the center of town. Expensive. Focus on seafood with an extensive wine list.

Gluten-free Ice Cream

Gelateria Porta Romana
Piazzale di Porta Romana
Tel: 055 221 121
Open: 11:00-13:45;15:00-24:00; closed Monday

Located about ten minutes from the Annalena entrance to the Boboli Gardens, this is one of the first ice cream parlors in town to offer delicious assorted gluten-free flavors in addition to their traditional homemade ice cream and frozen yogurt.

Resources

Following is a list of recent resources for Florence as well as for other major Italian cities. While much information is available in English, several major disability web sites in Italian with helpful information on tourism have also been included. If you do not read Italian, use *http://babelfish.altavista.com* for translation. The list does not pretend to be all-inclusive but aims to give you the most useful tools, whenever possible in English, for planning a trip to Italy. Many sites provide links for additional information.

Ferrara

Surrounded by much of its Renaissance-fortified walls, Ferrara has a picturesque historic center with a medieval castle and some interesting Renaissance palaces. Just over an hour by fast Eurostar train, Ferrara is an easy day trip from Florence. There is accessible public bus transportation from the RR station to the center of town.

Tourist Information Office
Ufficio Informazioni e Accoglienza Turistica
Corso Giovecca, 21
44100 Ferrara
Tel: 0532 209 370
Fax: 0532 212 266
E-mail: *infotour@comune.fe.it*

Internet

www.comune.fe.it/turismo: For information on wheelchair accessibility, click on "10 itinerari per conoscere Ferrara," then on individual monuments, then on the international disability symbol.

www.ferraraterraeacqua.it: For general tourist information in English.

Mobility Center
Via Kennedy, 6
Tel: 0532 767 023
Open: Monday-Sunday, 9:00-18:00; closed on Thursday

Description: Has manual and power wheelchairs, scooters, and handy bikes for hire at €5,00 per day. Using this service also entitles you to free entrance to civic museums, with 15 percent discount in selected restaurants and 20 percent discount in selected hotels.

Publications

The publications below, available from the tourist information office, include information regarding wheelchair accessibility.

- *Six Routes to Love Ferrara*—proposes six itineraries for visiting the city.
- *Ferrara's Walls*—guidebook to the city's fifteenth-century fortified walls.
- *Ferrara*—multilingual tourist map gives indication of accessibility of hotels, pharmacies, public buildings, theaters, and historical monuments.

Fiesole

www.fiesolefacile.it (In Italian) A serious attempt to give accurate accessibility information on the town of Fiesole and its surrounding communities. Of special interest for tourists is the information on accommodations, places to eat, churches, and museums.

Florence

Barrier Free Travel
250 West 57th Street, Suite 916
New York, New York 10107

Via Benedetto da Foiano, 19
50125 Florence
Tel/Fax: 055 233 6128
E-mail: *barrierfreetravel@tin.it*

Description: An American nonprofit organization with official recognition in Italy, Barrier Free Travel has been active for five years in promoting accessible tourism in Florence and Tuscany through its publications, speaking engagements and general advocacy of travel for people with disabilities. Public funding and private contributions help support the organization's activities.

Barrier Free Travel Services
Via Benedetto da Foiano, 19
50125 Florence
Tel/Fax: 055 233 6128
E-mail: *info@bftservices.it*
Home Page: *www.bftservices.it*

Description: Barrier Free Travel Services opened its doors in 2004 to provide professional tour guide and consulting services to travelers with disabilities. In collaboration with select local tour operators BFT can also assist in planning trips in Florence and Tuscany, both for individuals and groups.

Internet

www.comune.firenze.it is the official site of the city of Florence. Good for general information. Click on "Vivere Firenze" for wheelchair-accessible itineraries (presently in Italian only). A printed version is available in English, see "Recent Publications" below.

www.firenzeturismo.it is the APT (Azienda per il Turismo di Firenze) or official city tourist board site.

www.turismo.toscana.it is the official site of the Regione Toscana.

Recent Publications

The Florence Experience. Tour Itineraries with Supplementary Information for the Disabled. This publication is part of the project *Vivere Firenze,* the city of Florence's most recent initiative concerning visitors with disabilities. A series of four guidebooks will describe four itineraries in the historical center which have been specifically designed for people in wheelchairs or with visual impairments. The itineraries include a historical description as well as guidelines for orientation and mobility. Each itinerary begins in Piazza della Repubblica, progresses in a counterclockwise direction, and can be completed in three hours. The first itinerary was published in 2003 and includes Piazza della Signoria, Piazzale degli Uffizi, Ponte Vecchio, Piazza Pitti, Ponte and Piazza Santa Trinita back to Piazza della Reppublica. Locations of a few pharmacies, wheelchair-accessible restrooms, and parking spaces are indicated. The second itinerary, published in 2004 (at the time of publication in Italian only), describes the neighborhood of Santa Maria Novella. An audiocassette of the first itinerary is also available (presently, in Italian only). You can find the printed guides and cassettes at tourist information centers.

Mappa dell'Accessibilità Urbana

This map, published by the city of Florence in 2000 for the Jubilee Year, indicates wheelchair-accessible pedestrian routes and reserved accessible parking places within the historic center. The accompanying pamphlet (*Guida alle Strutture e ai Servizi della Città*) is available in Italian only. Information given in the pamphlet is not always accurate, and the map tends to overestimate the city's true state of accessibility, and it is important to remember always to use extreme caution when navigating over Florence's stone-paved sidewalks and streets. Although the map and pamphlet have not been reprinted, copies should still be available at most tourist information centers with the exception of the airport.

Genoa

Terra di Mare
Piazza Matteotti, 72/r
Genova
Tel: 010 542 098
Open: Tuesday-Saturday, 9:00-13:00; 14:00-18:00
E-mail: *info@terradimare.it*
Home Page: *www.terradimare.it* (in Italian only)

Description: This tourist information bureau for visitors with disabilities gives information for Genoa and other towns in Liguria on lodging, places to eat, artistic monuments, and suggested wheelchair-accessible itineraries. Their database includes listings for 64 hotels and 180 restaurants. For information contact directly. Click on "Mobility Service" to reserve the loan of a four-wheel scooter while visiting Genoa.

Milan

AIAS
Sportello Vacanze Disabili
Via San Barnaba, 29
20122 Milano
Tel: 02 6765 4740
Fax: 02 5501 4870
E-mail: *aiasmi.vacanze@tiscalinet.it*
Home Page: *www.milanopertutti.it*

Description: This very informative web site has an extensive and reliable database of information, also in English, not only on accessible lodging, but also on accessible restaurants, museums, monuments, theaters, cinemas, pharmacies, shops, and transportation (via plane, train, subway, bus, taxi, automobile) in the greater Milan area.

Comments: The tourist information bureau of AIAS (Associazione Italiana Assistenza Spastici) prefers to answer questions in English by e-mail, letter, or fax. Be as specific as possible in your requests.

Rome and Lazio

CO.IN. (Consorzio Cooperative Integrate)
Via Enrico Giglioli, 54/a
00169 Roma
Tel: 06 712 9011
Fax: 06 7129 0179
E-mail: *turismo@coinsociale.it*
Home Page: *www.coinsociale.it (In English)* Gives information compiled by CO.IN. on accessible hotels, restaurants and cafés, museums and monuments, theaters, public restrooms, and transportation in Rome.

Description: CO.IN. has been active for over fifteen years on multiple disability issues on both national and European levels. Their tourist bureau supplies information on accessibility not only for Rome, but also for Italy in general. In addition, CO.IN. can provide adapted vans with drivers for hire for day trips or airport transfers and offers guided tours (also accessible to wheelchair users) to some of the major sites in and near Rome. These tours, which are very popular, have a long waiting list with priority given to city residents. See *www.romapertutti.it* (in Italian). Under "Visite guidate" you'll find a list of itineraries for the guided accessible tours offered by CO.IN. The following publications, compiled several years ago, are available directly from CO.IN. (they will not mail).

- *Giubileo Accessible.* Published in 2000 in occasion of the Jubilee Year. The maps are helpful, but information is limited to areas around the seven basilicas of Rome, including St. Peters, St. John the Lateran, and Santa Maria Maggiore.

- *Roma Accessible. Guida turistica per persone con disabilità, 1999* (multilingual). Published by CO.IN. in collaboration with the Department of Social Policies of the city of Rome. Information is divided by geographic area and includes lists of accessible hotels and restaurants, churches, museums, shopping, transportation, and other services.
- *Roma Perché no?/ Rome Why not?* (in Italian and English) A practical miniguide to accessible Rome giving general information on accessible transportation within Italy. Published prior to 1999.
- *Natura accessible: Parchi e riserve naturali del Lazio.* Two maps (Part 1, published in 1995; Part 2, in 1996) describing the accessibility of Lazio's major parks and natural reserves.

Lazio

In addition to the maps listed above by CO.IN. see *www.presidiolazio.it* (in Italian). Gives information on Lazio, the region in which Rome is located. By clicking on "Itinerari," then on "la Roma Archeologica" you'll find descriptions of an accessible itineraries through Trajan's Market and the Imperial Forum, including some useful photographs of the ramps and routes along the way.

Siena

www.comune.siena.it/turismo (also in English). Click on "Siena enabled" for useful information on parking, wheelchair access to museums, hotels, restaurants. Under general categories such as "Accommodations" or "Eating in Siena" to find a list of accessible places, click on "access for disabled people."

www.comune.siena.it/disabinf/access.html (in Italian) For some additional information on accessible hotels, restaurants, museums, cinemas and theaters, banks and parking in the town of Siena, including some other lodgings for "agriturismo" or farm holidays in the immediate surroundings.

Venice

Informahandicap

Viale Garibaldi, 155
30174 Mestre
Tel: 041 534 1700
Fax: 041 534 2257
E-mail: *informahandicap@comune.venezia.it*
Home Page: *www.comune.venezia.it/handicap/tourism*
Open: Tuesday, Thursday, 15:30-18:30; Tuesday, Friday 9:00-13:00

Description: A local organization for people with disabilities which can provide tourist information. Much of the information on the web site, including a description of the accessibility map to Venice, transportation, and places to eat, is also available in English.

Other

www.disabili.com
One of the major Italian sites on disability issues, giving some useful information on accessible tourism. Click on "Vacanze per tutti," "Musei," and "Tempo Libero" for all kinds of suggestions including a list of *agriturismi* (farm holiday) listings all over Italy, and depending on the season, ideas for special ski vacations and ski instruction in the Italian Alps or holidays at the beach. There is also a list of Italian travel agencies and tour operators to help you plan your accessible vacation, although some tend to be expensive and not always 100 percent reliable.

www.italiapertutti.it
A project sponsored by the Italian government Department of Tourism to survey hotels, restaurants, and other tourist-oriented structures nationwide for accessibility information. Not all of the site information is available in English, nor does much new information seem to have been added since the project was launched in 1999.

www.superabile.it
This serious and comprehensive site is sponsored by INAIL (*Istituto Nazionale per l'Assicurazione contro gli Infortuni sul Lavoro* or National Institute for Insurance Against Work Injuries). By clicking on "Tempo Libero" and then "Vacanze Info Point" you will find a list of published tour guides, national tourist information bureaus, and some proposals for vacations for people with disabilities. There is also a useful search engine for locating accessible accommodations in Milan and Rome.

Barrier Free Travel. A Nuts and Bolts Guide for Wheelers and Slow Walkers by Candy Harrington, published in 2001 by Xlibris. Although this publication deals primarily with taking a trip within the USA, it gives useful tips on travel in general, including infomation on taking a plane and how to deal with travel agents in planning your trip; an indispensable guide to anyone who wants to do it on their own.

Turismo senza barriere (Milan, 2004), published by the Italian Touring Club, is a guide to select museums, monuments, national parks, sports activities, places to eat, and accomodations located throughout Italy and chosen for their high accessibility rating. Available in Italian only, this small, new guide also includes a useful section on resources.

English to Italian Glossary of Useful Access Words and Phrases

General

disabled. *Disabile.* The term *handicappato(a)* is used less frequently.
I am disabled. *Sono una persona disabile.*
I use a wheelchair. *Uso una sedia a rotelle.*
I use a power wheelchair. *Uso una carrozzina elettronica.*
I am unable to walk very far. *Non posso camminare . . . molto lontano.*
blind. *Non vedente. Cieco(a)* is used less frequently.
I am blind. *Sono non vedente.*
Braille. The same word is used in Italian, pronounced "brile" (with a long *i* and silent *e* like "pile").
guide dog. *Cane guida.*
deaf. *Non udente / sordo(a)* is used less frequently.
I am deaf. *Sono non udente. Sono sordo.*
hearing impaired. *Ipoudente.*
I am hearing impaired. I don't hear well. *Sono ipoudente. Sono quasi sordo.*
sign language. *Linguaggio dei sordomuti.*
sign language interpreter. *Un interprete del linguaggio dei sordomuti.*

Wheelchairs

wheelchair. *Sedia a rotelle* or *carrozzella* or *carrozzina.*
wheel. *Ruota.*
tire. *Gomma.*
battery. *Batteria.*

battery charger. *Caricabatteria.*
circuit breaker. *Fusibile.*
My wheelchair needs to be repaired. *La mia sedia a rotelle ha bisogno di essere riparata.*

Equipment

cane. *Bastone.*
crutches. *Gruccie.*
ramp. *Rampa. Scivolo. Pedana.*
transfer board. *Tavoletta di trasferimento.*
wheelchair lift (van/bus). *Sollevatore.*

Stairs and Elevators

elevator. *Ascensore.*
stairlift. *Servoscala* or *Montascale.*
stairs. *Scale.*
Are there stairs? *Ci sono delle scale?*
How many flights of stairs/steps are there? *Quante rampe di scale ci sono? Quanti gradini sono?*
Is there an entrance without stairs/steps? *C'è un ingresso senza scale . . . senza gradini?*
Is there a ramp? *C'è una rampa?* or . . . *uno scivolo?* Or . . . *una pedana?*
Is there an elevator? *C'è un ascensore?*
Where is the elevator? *Dove si trova l'ascensore?*
Is it necessary to climb any stairs to get to the elevator? *Ci sono dei gradini per arrivare all'ascensore?*
What are the elevator's dimensions? *Quali sono le dimensioni dell'ascensore?*
What is the width? *Quanto è largo?*
What is the depth? *Quanto è profondo?*
What is the width of the doorway? *Qual' è la largezza della porta?*
The elevator/ramp/platform lift is broken. *L'ascensore/ la rampa/il sollevatore è rotto* (or *rotta* depending on the gender of the noun).

Bedrooms and Bathrooms

What is the height of the bed? *Qual' è l'altezza del letto?*
accessible bathroom. *Bagno (or "servizio igenico") accessible.*
Is the bathroom wheelchair accessible? *Il bagno è accessible alle sedie a rotelle?*
grab bars. *Maniglioni.*
retractable grab bar. *Maniglione ribaltabile.*
handrails. *Corrimani.*
roll-in shower. *Doccia a pavimento.*
Does the bathroom have a roll-in shower? *Il bagno è con doccia a pavimento?*
Are there grab bars in the bathroom/in the shower/next to the toilet? *Ci sono dei maniglioni nel bagno/nella doccia/accanto al wc?*
(pronounced "voo ci")
Is there a shower bench? *C'è un sedile nella doccia?*
retractable shower bench. *Sedile ribaltabile.*

Directions

up. *Su.*
down. *Giù.*
right. *Destra.*
left. *Sinistra.*
Turn right/left. *Girare a destra/ a sinistra.*
How far is it from (—) to (—)? *Quanto dista* (Firenze) *da* (Siena)?
How many kilometers is it to (Siena)? *Quanti kilometri ci sono per andare a* (Siena)?
How many meters is it to the entrance? *Quanti metri ci sono fino all'ingresso?*
How far is it from the bus stop to the entrance of the museum? *Quanto c'è dalla fermata dell'autobus fino all'ingresso del museo?*

Transportation

Is the bus wheelchair accessible? *L'autobus è accessibile alle sedie a rotelle?*

Is the bus stop accessible? *È accessibile la fermata dell'autobus?* **next stop.** *La prossima fermata.*
Is the train wheelchair accessible? *Il treno è accessibile alle sedie a rotelle?*
Is the van/minivan wheelchair accessible? *Il pulmino è accessibile alle sedie a rotelle?*
Does the van have a ramp? *Il pulmino ha una rampa?*
Does the van have a lift? *Il pulmino ha un sollevatore?*
Do you have an adapted car/van for hire with hand controls? *Ha in noleggio una macchina allestita /un pulmino allestito/ con controlli a mano?*
Do you have a car with automatic shift for hire? *Ha una macchina in noleggio con cambio automatico?*

Pronunciation Guide

Every letter (vowel and consonant) is pronounced in Italian. There is no silent *e*, for example, as there is in English.

A is always a short *a* (as in "adopt")
E sounds like a long *a* (as in "ate")
I sounds like a long *e* (as in "eat")
O sounds like a long *o* (as in "oats")
U sounds like *oo* (as in "too")
C has a hard sound like *k* before *u, o* and *a* (*carrozzella*) *but before other vowels* it sounds like the "ch" in "chair" (*doccia*)

Rules of Gender Agreement

Masculine and feminine gender agreement, as in French or Spanish, is also used in Italian.
Masculine gender endings are *o* (singular) and *i* (plural).
Example: *corrimano, corrimani* (handrail/s)
Feminine gender endings are *a* (singular) and *e* (plural).
Example: *rampa, rampe* (ramp/s)
There are the inevitable exceptions to the rule. Some words in singular form end in *e* and in plural in *i* for both masculine and feminine forms.
Example: *interprete, interpreti* (interpreter/s)

Conversion to the Metric System

Basic measurements of length, area, liquids, weights, and temperatures have been listed below together with some shortcut methods for easier remembering day to day as you plan what to wear according to local temperature, purchase gas, or buy picnic cold cuts from the grocer. It is best to use exact measurements when calculating the weight and size of your wheelchair, especially for stair lift information as US stair lifts tend to be slightly larger and capable of carrying more weight.

Units of Length and Area

Standard
One inch = 2.54 centimeters
One centimeter = 0.3937 inches
One meter = 39.4 inches or 3 feet 3 inches
One square meter = 10.76 square feet
One kilometer = 0.621 miles
One mile = 1.61 kilometers
One acre = 0.4047 hectares

Shortcuts
One inch = 2.5 centimeters
Four inches = 10 centimeters
One foot = 30 centimeters
One meter = just over a yard
One kilometer = $^5/_8$ mile
Three kilometers = almost 2 miles
One hectare = 2.5 acres

Basic measurements of interest to wheelchair and scooter users:

According to Italian law governing architecture barriers, exterior doors should measure 80 centimeters (31 ½ inches); interior doors: 75 centimeters (29 ½ inches), with maximum rise at a threshold of 2.5 centimeters (1 inch). You may find in newer constructions that doors may be as wide as 90 centimeters (35 ½ inches).

Units of Weight

Standard
One pound = 0.4536 kg (kilograms)
One kilogram = 2.2046 pounds

Shortcuts
One pound = just under ½ kilogram
One kilogram = 2.2 pounds
One hundred grams (In Italian also known as an *etto*) = just under ¼ pound

Two hundred and fifty grams = just over ½ pound (for example *due etti e mezzo di prosciutto [250 grams]* = just over ½ pound of sliced ham).

Units of Liquid Measure

Standard
One liter = 1.056 US liquid quarts/0.8880 English quarts
One liter = 0.264 US gallon/0.220 English gallon

Shortcuts
One quart = just under one liter
One US gallon = just under 4 liters. (By dividing the number of liters of gas you purchase by 4, you will know the approximate equivalent in US gallons.

Temperature

Standard
Fahrenheit to Centigrade (also known as Celsius): subtract 32, multiply by 5, divide by 9
Centigrade to Fahrenheit: multiply by 9, divide by 5, add 32
Water freezes at 0° C = 32° F
Water boils at 100° C = 212° F
Normal body temperature 98.6° F = 37° C

Shortcuts
To convert Centigrade to Fahrenheit: double the amount in centigrade and add 30
(For example: 20° C = 20+20+30 = 70° F)

To convert Fahrenheit to Centigrade: subtract 30 and divide the result in half
(For example, 90° F = 90-30 = 60 divided by 2 = 30° C)

Printed in the United States
117468LV00003B/86/A